Going Against the Grain

How Reducing and Avoiding Grains Can Revitalize Your Health

Melissa Diane Smith

Contemporary Books

Chicago   New York   San Francisco   Lisbon   London   Madrid   Mexico City
Milan   New Delhi   San Juan   Seoul   Singapore   Sydney   Toronto

Library of Congress Cataloging-in-Publication Data

Smith, Melissa Diane.
    Going against the grain: how reducing and avoiding grain can revitalize your health /
    Melissa Diane Smith.
       p. cm.
    Includes bibliographical references and index.
    ISBN 0-658-01722-5
    1. Low-carbohydrate diet. 2. Grain—Toxicology. 3. Gluten-free diet
    4. Malabsorption syndromes—Diet therapy.   I. Title.

    RM237.73 .S63 2002
    613.2'83—dc21   2001056063

Contemporary Books

*A Division of The **McGraw·Hill** Companies*

3   4   5   6   7   8   9   10   DOC/DOC   1   10   9   8   7   6   5   4   3   2

International Standard Book Number: 0-658-01722-5

This book was set in Berkeley by Kate Mueller.
Printed and bound by R. R. Donnelley—Crawfordsville

Cover design by Mike Stromberg / The Great American Art Co.
Interior design by Kate Mueller / Electric Dragon Productions

McGraw-Hill Books are available at special quantity discounts to use as premiums and sales promotions, or for use in corporate training programs. For more information, please write to the Director of Special Sales, Professional Publishing, McGraw-Hill, Two Penn Plaza, New York, NY 10121-2998. Or contact your local bookstore.

The purpose of this book is to educate. It is sold with the understanding that the publisher and author shall have neither liability nor responsibility for any injury caused or alleged to be caused directly or indirectly by the information contained in this book. While every effort has been made to ensure its accuracy, the book's contents should not be construed as medical advice. Each person's health needs are unique. To obtain recommendations appropriate to your particular situation, please consult a qualified health care provider.

This book is dedicated to
Helen and Don, incredible people
who just happen to be my parents;
the grandmother I never knew; and
all the people who can benefit
from this message.

Praise for *Going Against the Grain*

"Melissa Diane Smith has courageously and accurately tackled what has emerged as America's primary food-related health problem: disease and obesity attributable to the regular consumption of high-calorie, nutrient-poor, immune-disruptive grains. I applaud her effort. This is a must-read book for the health-conscious person wanting to maintain health, as well as for the disease-laden individual trying to regain health."
   —*Kenneth D. Fine, M.D., gluten sensitivity researcher and director of The Intestinal Health Institute, Dallas, Texas*

"A myth-breaking book that could transform the health and disease statistics of this country. Melissa Diane Smith's writing is clear, friendly, and persuasive. Everyone, including doctors, should read this book."
   —*Ralph Golan, M.D., author of* Optimal Wellness

"An intriguing book loaded with practical nutrition advice that you won't want to stop reading. Melissa Diane Smith is a gifted writer, and I am impressed with the work she has put into this book."
   —*Annemaria Ballin, Ph.D., founder and director of education, American Academy of Nutrition*

"A truly original and eye-opening book. Melissa Diane Smith destroys the myth that grains are the staff of life, while explaining how they make people sick. You, too, will want to go 'against the grain' in pursuit of good health."
   —*Jack Challem,* The Nutrition Reporter *and coauthor of* Syndrome X

"In this book, Melissa Diane Smith describes in excellent detail why a diet that goes against the grain is so good for so many."
   —*Abram Hoffer, M.D., Ph.D., nutritional medicine pioneer and author of eighteen nutrition books*

"Based on solid science, *Going Against the Grain* invites the reader to conduct an experiment in the laboratory of his own body, possibly to uncover a hidden key to otherwise unexplained symptoms and illness. I really like this book."
   —*Ron Hunninghake, M.D., medical director, the Center for the Improvement of Human Functioning*

"*Going Against the Grain* does a superb job of accurately pointing out potential health problems associated with eating grains. The book is lively, to the point, and transforms difficult scientific concepts into explanations that are easily understood. This information has been sorely needed by the public."
   —*Loren Cordain, Ph.D., Colorado State University health science professor and author of* The Paleo Diet

Contents

Acknowledgments

I had to go against the grain to sell and write this book. Fortunately, I had many supporters and unexpected angels who helped me make my labor of love become a reality. My most sincere thanks and gratitude go to:

- Mike Cohn, my literary agent, who worked with me to find a publishing home for this book

- Editor Claudia McCowan, who bought this idea; Dianne Woo, for development suggestions; Kate Mueller, for her illustration, design, and layout work; Garret Lemoi, who oversaw the editorial process; and Rena Copperman, who oversaw the production of this book

- My clients who have taught me so much with their candor and honesty

- The health professionals and scientists who inspired me with their work and graciously agreed to share ideas and information: James Braly, M.D.; Loren Cordain, Ph.D.; Alessio Fasano, M.D.; Kenneth Fine, M.D.; Laura Johnson-Kelly, M.A.; Ron Rosedale, M.D.; and Hunter Yost, M.D.

- Diane Perrine, who was very generous in sharing information on celiac disease and hidden forms of gluten with me; Liz Attanasio, who helped me with information in the eleventh hour; and Cynthia Kuper, R.D., and Elaine Monarch, who put me in touch with many celiacs to interview

- Lara Evans, Beth Salmon, Nicole Brechka, and Peggy Wagener, editors who signed on to my going-against-the-grain ideas long before others did

- Noelle Kuhn, Jill Ruttenberg, Ramesh Jagasia, Lawrence Lang, and Stuart Sandler, who were always willing to offer a supportive word (most especially Stuart who helped me go against the grain many years ago to regain my health)

- My two terrific brothers, Ron Smith and Rich Smith, and my father, Don Smith, whose steadfast belief in me and my ability to do this book meant so much to me

- Holly Sollars, a close friend and talented recipe developer and baker, who shared several memorable "bake-a-thon" days with me

- Mindie Jo Snyder, my creative, loving sister in spirit, who worked with me to develop the gluten sensitivity artistic concept

- Jack Challem, my colleague on many projects from E to X, who encouraged me to write the proposal for this book and offered me key suggestions, important research, and some of his savvy and experience in the health food industry and nutritional medicine field

- Most especially, Helen Caldes Smith, the best mother, supporter, cook, and copy editor anyone could ever ask for. I am eternally grateful for her help and support.

Last but not least, I must thank the great horned owl who hoot-hoot-hooted in the tree outside my place and kept me company when I worked late into the night. He, his mate, and their offspring gave me indescribable joy and inspiration and centered me in a way that only nature and wildlife can. As the baby owl was learning to fly, this book was finally getting its wings. That seemed like a powerful sign to keep going, so this book could fly, too.

Introduction

Grains may seem the staff of life, but they're really scythes that insidiously whittle away most people's health.

Although the U.S. government promotes a high intake of grains (such as pastas, breads, and cereals), following this strategy actually sets us up for health problems.

To stay fit and free of disease, all of us should eat fewer grains. Some of us should eat no grains at all.

If these statements contradict everything you've heard about diet, I can understand. More than a decade ago, they would have seemed radical to me as well—the antithesis of what I had been taught to believe. But experience and research have taught me that grains have an unrecognized—but very strong—dark side. Eating a lot of them can lead to virtually every one of the health problems plaguing North Americans today—including obesity, heart disease, diabetes, some types of cancer, fatigue, minor and serious digestive disorders, dementia, and psychological problems. To prevent these health complaints—and to feel and look our best—we need to understand the little-known dangers of grains, and then go against the grain of social pressure to avoid eating these foods morning, noon, and night.

In a society where wheat is eaten at almost every meal, pasta is promoted as a healthy food, and the heart of the continent is endearingly referred to as "the bread basket," it seems almost sacrilegious (or un-American) to speak out against grains. However, the research pointing to the health benefits of a low- to no-grain diet is simply too convincing to ignore. *Going Against the Grain* will cut through the hype you have come to believe and food companies want you to believe—that grains should be the centerpiece of your diet. Instead, this book will present convincing evidence that grains should play a minimal role in your diet.

Even if you presently eat a lot of grains and feel healthy, this book still has an important message for you. It will make you aware of the potential long-term dangers of an excessive intake of grains and will explain why a diet that favors vegetables over grains is the secret of success for long-term weight control and health.

What This Book Reveals

Here's a sampling of the nutrition insights this book reveals:

- Refined grains, such as pastas, breads, rolls, bagels, muffins, and most cereals, form the foundation of most Americans' diets. By loading up on these foods, you set yourself up for degenerative diseases such as heart disease and adult-onset diabetes.

- Whole grains, which are often recommended by many nutritionists in place of refined grains, have more nutrients than nutrient-stripped refined grains, but they also have many *anti*nutrients that inhibit nutrient absorption and interfere with health. Eating a lot of whole grains—something advocated by many health-food experts—can ultimately cause nutrient deficiencies and set the stage for such diseases as anemia, osteoporosis, and autoimmune disorders.

- Millions of people unknowingly have sensitivity to gluten, a protein in many common grains. Sometimes taking the form of "silent celiac disease," gluten sensitivity slowly erodes people's health, damages the intestinal tract, and greatly increases the risk for nutrient deficiencies, small intestine cancer, autoimmune diseases, and osteoporosis. Unlike people with classic celiac disease, who have obvious symptoms such as bloating, weight loss, and diarrhea, most people who have gluten sensitivity are asymptomatic or have very nonspecific, vague symptoms, such as fatigue, a nearly universal complaint.

- Grain allergies and addictions (especially to wheat) are exceedingly common, and they are unrecognized contributors to the growing epidemic of obesity. Like alcoholics, many people repeatedly eat foods they're allergic to at every meal to get a temporary "high" from drug-like compounds in them. When that feeling wears off, they crave another "fix" of the problem food to regain that euphoric feeling. Unrecognized grain allergies and addictions set the stage for just-got-to-have-it cravings, binge-eating, and overeating, which ultimately lead to weight gain.

If you've been socialized to believe grains are good for you (as virtually everybody in modern society has), this information may be a bit unsettling—it probably turns your belief system upside down. (It might sound like I'm saying, "The sky is green, and the grass is blue.") Don't worry, though. You have in your hands the one book that will take you step by step through what you need to know to gradually change your belief system and your actions to go against the grain and revitalize your health.

Why should I debunk the status quo message sung by mainstream doctors and dietitians for decades? It's high time someone did. No one else seems to be speaking out on this topic, and the health of North Americans is suffering in the process. More important, my firsthand experience has convinced me of the need to stand up to critics and go against the grain of conventional dietary wisdom.

My Story

Fifteen years ago, I worked at a world-famous health resort known for its ability to transform overweight guests into slimmer and presumably healthier people. As a public relations writer for the spa, I wrote stories that educated and inspired guests and employees about the value of the low-fat, high-carbohydrate, grain-rich diet. This was a health prescription I believed was beneficial for everyone, but my personal and professional experiences since then have drastically altered my views about nutrition. They have led me to the surprising but inescapable conclusion that eating a high-grain diet is hazardous to most people's health over the long term.

In retrospect, I should have recognized the signs warning me I didn't thrive on a high-grain diet. For one thing, I was just plain hungry much of the time. I didn't want to lose my trim figure though, so I tried to ignore my hunger pangs and kept a tight rein on what I ate. Other warning signs appeared. Less than a year into my job at the spa, I came down with a series of viruses and strep throat infections. Six months later, I looked puffy and started to gain weight. Although I was not eating much food, I found it increasingly difficult to fit into my size 6 skirts and slacks and eventually outgrew them altogether. In addition, I—the editor of the health resort's employee newsletter—always had been an organized thinker with a sharp mind, but I often had trouble remembering if a story had been written or even if I had assigned it to someone!

It never once occurred to me that my diet could be contributing to my health problems. I paid dearly for this naïveté. Labor Day weekend of 1987 I developed a very severe, mysterious, flulike illness (much later diagnosed as chronic fatigue syndrome) that I could not shake. I then began a five-year odyssey in which I desperately searched for answers and solutions for my health problems. After seeing a series of doctors who were baffled by my condition and unable to help me, I turned in desperation to nutrition. At first I tried eating what I thought were healthful foods, especially vegetarian, macrobiotic, and other meals centered around grains. But the more I ate light foods—something virtually everyone in nutrition advocated at the time—the more my health worsened. I experienced an aggravation of my sore throats, increased digestive discomfort and bloating, depression, and greater difficulty getting out of bed each morning. Perhaps even more shocking to me was the lighter I ate, the heavier I became. By spring of 1988, I had ballooned to 145 pounds and found myself having to buy a size 13 pair of pants because none of my other clothes fit me!

Frustrated beyond belief, I delved further into nutrition books and health magazines and decided to try a radical new strategy: a wheat-free, hypoallergenic diet rich in lean animal protein and lots of vegetables. Going against the grain of prevailing nutritional wisdom and the spa-type diet I believed in was a challenge, but a strange—and wonderful—thing happened during my experiment: I started to gradually, *effortlessly* lose fat. I didn't understand why but was elated with this development and stuck with the diet, difficult as it seemed. After about six months, I lost all the weight I had gained and was back to 115 pounds.

I wasn't entirely free of chronic fatigue syndrome, but because I had regained my slim figure, I thought I could go off my diet. What a mistake! I didn't understand then that a diet low in grains was actually the food plan I needed for optimal, long-term health.

Naturally, I wanted to add wheat back to my diet, not only because everyone in America was eating wheat but also because I was literally crazy about it before I started my therapeutic diet. I thought as long as I avoided nutrient-stripped white-flour products and ate only whole grains, I could add wheat back. What I discovered, though, again surprised me. I found that when I ate wheat after avoiding it for a long time, I initially felt euphoric and wanted to binge on it. A day later, though, I felt even more tired, sick, and depressed than usual and was plagued by digestive problems. Through trial and error, I eventually found similar unpleasant reactions after I ate oats and other gluten-containing grains, such as rye, barley, spelt and kamut.

This experience frustrated me once again. On the one hand, I had stumbled on a diet that was truly therapeutic for me—a diet that was enabling me to recover from chronic fatigue syndrome when nothing else could. I was feeling and looking good, better than I had in years. Everything indicated that following this diet was my best shot to conquer my sickness. On the other hand, I wanted desperately to be "normal" and *not* go against the grain. I wanted to eat and be like everybody else and not be weird or make waves or stand out like a sore thumb. A real tug-of-war was going on inside me.

Fortunately, my desire for health won out. Although I certainly had my setbacks, occasionally succumbing to the tremendous pressure in our grain-obsessed world, the fact that I felt so lousy after eating grains kept me on the straight and narrow as time went on. The seriousness of chronic fatigue syndrome forced me to persist on a diet that went against the grain (at least the gluten grains), and this was a blessing in disguise. My diet not only allowed me to regain my health but to maintain it ever since.

The Stories of Others

Despite my success with a gluten-free, low-grain diet, I didn't talk about it much. I was actually a bit embarrassed and thought I was just one weird exception to the rule that high-grain diets were good for people. That idea changed, though, after I received my nutrition education from the American Academy of Nutrition and became a nutrition counselor.

When I first started to counsel people, most of my clients complained about gaining weight even though they were following the widely promoted low-fat, high-carbohydrate, high-grain diet to a T. This refrain sounded very familiar to me, so I advised them to cut down on grains (especially wheat) and instead eat more vegetables. One by one, over and over again, my clients came back telling me how pleased they were with this strategy. As long as they followed this way of eating, they lost both fat and water weight, trimmed down (especially through the middle), and often had digestive complaints clear up or a lessening of heart disease risk factors, such as a reduction of high blood pressure, cholesterol, or triglycerides. These results were dramatic!

However, my clients complained about how hard it was to keep eating this way, especially when they were eating out, because they encountered wheat-based foods at every turn. "Isn't there some way I can go back to my old way of eating and get the same health results?" they would plead. I would relay my experience and the experiences of other clients—that eating a lot of grains subtly degraded health—and convince them to stick with the low-grain diet. Then I would spend most of my time counseling them on the *practical* ways they could keep going against the grain for their health while still leading as normal and sociable a life as possible.

My professional experience as a nutrition counselor and my personal experience were not the only things that shaped my strong belief in the widespread health benefits of a low-grain diet. As a health journalist, I have interviewed dozens of physicians and nutrition professionals who have witnessed the same dramatic results with low-grain diets, and I have seen a wealth of scientific studies pile up about the health hazards of grains. From all fronts, the message has been getting louder and louder to speak out and let the world know about the importance of going against the grain for health. I heard the call, and that's what this book is all about.

In Chapters 1 and 2, you'll learn how we've been seduced into eating an excess of grains, even though the diet we were designed for contained few or no grains. The next four chapters will give you cutting-edge information about the many nutritional problems with grains and the types of health complaints these problems can lead to. The second half of the book will help you identify your individual sensitivity to grains and the type of against-the-grain diet that is best for you. It will also provide original menu plans, recipes, and eating out suggestions, so that you can go against the grain with minimal effort and hassle.

No matter what your health concern is—whether you are trying to lose weight, fend off fatigue and digestive bloating, or simply prevent heart disease or diabetes—do yourself a favor and sit back and delve into this book. If you use the book to help you go against the grain (to the degree that's best for you), I'm confident you will substantially reduce your risks for numerous age-related degenerative diseases and find yourself looking and feeling better than you have in years.

THE PROBLEMS WITH GRAINS

CHAPTER 1

Grain Gluttony and Grain-O-Mania

Grain gluttony and grain-o-mania have overtaken our nation. So pervasive are grains in our diet that many of us don't realize we're eating grains in different forms every day, usually at every meal. Think cereal, toast or bagels for breakfast . . . sandwiches for lunch . . . muffins, doughnuts, or cookies for coffee breaks . . . pretzels or corn chips for snacks . . . pasta, pizza, or Mexican food for dinner. What's more, many of us don't eat just small portions of grain-based foods. We long for more and more of these foods and end up eating way too many of them. Grain-o-mania, therefore, is an excessive, persistent enthusiasm, interest, liking, or craving for grains, and grain gluttony is eating grains with abandon, especially habitually.

Grain-o-mania is so common that most people find it hard to imagine life without grains. Grain-o-maniacs get so much pleasure out of grains that they share stories of "to-die-for" croissants at one restaurant, "addictive" cornbread at another restaurant, and "awesome" fettucini and tortellini at a third. Grain gluttony goes hand in hand with grain-o-mania and is so accepted in our society that most people don't think it's unusual to truly "pig out" on grains. Grain gluttons love restaurants that have never-ending pasta bowls and all-you-can-eat Chinese food. They stuff their faces, then go back for one, two, three, or four more helpings.

Grain-o-mania

an excessive, persistent enthusiasm, interest, liking, or craving for grains

Grain gluttony

"pigging out" on grains, especially habitually

What's Wrong with a High Intake of Grains?

You may think there's nothing wrong with loading up on grains. After all, grains are good for us, aren't they? Well, no, that's a common misconception. The surprising truth is that grains aren't good for any of us in large amounts, and for some of us, they aren't good in any amounts at all. You'll learn all about these revelations in future chapters, but here are a few basics:

- Grains are high in carbohydrates and high in calories, especially when compared to the nutrients they provide.

- Grains are used to fatten up livestock, and they do the same to us when we eat them in excess.

- Millions of people are intolerant to common grains and develop allergic symptoms; aches and pains; malabsorption of nutrients; and/or bloating, gas, and other digestive upsets from eating them.

- High-grain diets are associated with, or implicated in, most modern-day health problems—everything from bone diseases, such as osteoporosis, to autoimmune diseases, such as autoimmune thyroid disease, to the major killers of today, such as heart disease, Type 2 diabetes, and some types of cancer.

Factors That Have Led to a High Intake of Grains

Naturally, you may be wondering: if grains aren't that good for us, why do most of us believe they are? And why have grains become such a major focus of our day-to-day attention, desire, and diets? Well, the answers to those questions are complicated. There are many pieces to the puzzle.

Availability, Social Programming, Advertising, and Promotions

First, grains are everywhere in our society: they permeate the culture on all levels and in all places. Grains are found in many shapes and forms at every restaurant, supermarket, food court, and concession stand. Think about the omnipresent complimentary bread basket in restaurants; the thousands of products that line the inner aisles of supermarkets; the supersize pretzels and cookies in shopping mall food courts; and the nachos, pizza, and beer offered at sporting events. Wherever we go, even on plane rides or boat cruises, grains are there: they show up as mystery snack mixes, muffins, sandwiches, and pasta dishes. Because grains are so available, most of us end up eating them out of sheer convenience if nothing else—even if we don't realize it or really want to.

Second, we've been socialized to believe that grains are good for us. We grew up learning that grains were one of the four major food groups essential to a balanced diet, at least as important as fruits and vegetables and more important than meat. In more recent years, we've heard about the food pyramid guideline, which makes grains the most important food group and suggests an unrealistic intake of six to eleven servings of grains per day. These guidelines have seeped into early grade-school education and the media's coverage of health stories. We, in turn, keep hearing the message, whether it's in the background or the foreground. So, for most of us, it's a given that grains are important foods, and we should eat a lot of them. Few of us have had the opportunity to hear any negatives about grains, so few question the grains-are-good idea. Even if we do question it, we reason that because everyone believes this, it must be true.

Third, food manufacturers, supermarkets, and restaurants offer us many incentives to eat a lot of grains. That's because grain-based foods have long shelf lives, can be twisted into virtually any shape or form imaginable, and are cheap to make. Food purveyors, therefore, love to push these foods because they can mark them up for a huge profit and make a lot of money. For example, bread is made from about five cents of wheat, but it usually sells for one to four dollars a loaf. Supermarkets and bakeries then sometimes give us coupons or "special prices" to make us think we're getting a deal by buying the bread. Similar promotions occur with cereal and other grain products. Advertisers also up the ante by running ads for cereals and breads that use warm and fuzzy terms such as "full of hearty grains and country goodness" and "farm-fresh bread": they know how to appeal to our inner desire for fresh, wholesome foods, even if that's not what we're really getting.

The Addictive Nature of Grains

These factors encourage us to eat a lot of grains, then we get hooked. We begin to feel like we need grain products. That's because the most common grain-based foods we eat provoke blood sugar highs often followed by blood sugar lows. Those blood sugar lows leave us yearning for a quick fix of energy a few hours later. Because grain products are readily available anywhere we go and most raise blood sugar quickly, we eat grains (often combined with sugar or other sweeteners) to temporarily solve our lagging energy brought about by imbalanced blood sugar.

But that's not the only way we get hooked. Grains have druglike substances that create true food addictions and cravings in some, if not many, people. Eating grains can promote at least a sense of comfort and sometimes a high or euphoric feeling. (You'll learn about this in detail in Chapter 6). A typical scenario is this: We eat grains in different forms every few hours without realizing it, first because it's the handy thing to do, then, as time goes on, to satisfy our cravings and to get our "hits" so we can temporarily feel good or avoid feeling bad. At that point, we are grain junkies, true habitual users of grains. We can't get off them and we pay for this in the long run. This isn't much different than kids who try smoking when they're young and impressionable, then start to psychologically and physically need cigarettes and become regular smokers. The only difference is that the habit of smoking isn't as accepted today as grain-o-mania and grain gluttony are.

The grain industry seems to be well aware of the addictive nature of grains (particularly combined with sweeteners)—or at least it knows which foods are selling like wildfire—and it tries to use this to its advantage. A vivid image that sticks in my mind is a cartoon of kids chowing down on Oreo cookies, saying, "Wow, these things are addictive!" Behind them, a father sits reading a newspaper story about Philip Morris, the big cigarette manufacturer, buying the maker of Oreos. Philip Morris, now the largest food manufacturer in the world, is changing its name to Altria and trying hard to look socially responsible these days by making philanthropic contributions. But the company is really involved in making money off people's addictions. The Philip Morris family of companies includes not only Kraft Foods and Nabisco Foods, makers of a number of cookies, cereals, and snack foods, but also the Post Cereal Company and the Miller beer company. These companies manufacture a wide variety of habit-forming, grain-based foods. Jack Challem, the coauthor of my previous book, *Syndrome X*, refers to Philip Morris as "Addiction, Inc.," which seems very fitting. Indeed, the name Altria is adapted from the Latin word *altus*, which means "high."

Food manufacturers and retailers know that children who become hooked on grains become adults who stay hooked on grains. So, they increasingly use clever promotions to influence impressionable kids into eating a lot of grain-based foods and equating grain-based foods with fun and entertainment. For example, fast-food restaurants, which are built around burgers with buns and high-fructose corn-syrup sweetened soft drinks, offer limited-time-only toys associated with the latest popular movie. Kids get their parents to bring them in for the toys, the whole family loads up on the food and drinks, and the kids develop a loyalty to fast-food restaurants from an early age. Another common promotion that appeals to children is putting toys in boxes of cereals and grain-based snack foods such as Cracker Jack. (As a child, I hated Cracker Jack, but used to beg my mom to buy it for me so I could get the toy inside!)

The latest programming-kids-early schemes are amusement parks that center around cereal characters and themes—Cereal City, USA, by

Kellogg's in Battle Creek, Michigan, and Cereal Adventure by General Mills in Bloomington, Minnesota. By walking down the Wheaties Hall of Champions and playing in the Lucky Charms Magical Forest, kids will develop an allegiance to cereals and specific brands early in life and, the manufacturers hope, will then become consumers for life.

The Consequences of Grain Gluttony and Grain-O-Mania

So, through a very complicated interplay between social programming, advertising, education, special promotions, and the habit-forming characteristics of grain-based foods, grain gluttony and grain-o-mania have now become everyday occurrences. As a result of all these clever promotions, cereal is now children's main source of vitamins. Kids junk out on grain- and sugar-based foods nearly all day long, almost to the exclusion of nutritious foods, such as vegetables. Consequently, the incidence of obesity and Type 2 diabetes (also called adult-onset diabetes) in children is at an all-time high.

And the situation is even worse for adults, many of whom have been grain junkies for a lot longer. The overall incidence of diabetes among Americans increased by 33 percent from 1990 to 1998, and among people in their thirties, the incidence jumped by an astounding 70 percent! Furthermore, 61 percent of all Americans are now overweight. If something isn't done soon to correct this trend, it's estimated that everyone could be overweight by the year 2020. Diabetes and being overweight are just two of the most obvious problems caused by grain gluttony, but they are by no means the only ones, as you'll discover throughout this book.

In the next chapter, you'll learn how the grain gluttony of today is very different than the diet we were designed for. By taking a trip down food history lane, you'll finally get the straight scoop you haven't heard before: every time people have changed their diets to include more grains, they have developed worse health problems. If we load up on grains, we set ourselves up for countless diseases that humans didn't develop when they ate few or no grains.

CHAPTER 2

A Trip Down Food History Lane

Most people think it's natural to eat grains, but it's really not. If you were to step into a field of grain and take a few stalks and chew them, you wouldn't get much satisfaction. Grains in their natural state are tough and pretty much indigestible—dramatically different from the grain foods we know today.

So, how did grains come to be an everyday component of most diets throughout the world? No one knows for sure how it all began, but about 10,000 to 15,000 years ago, our distant ancestors in the Middle East learned that grains needed to be processed in various ways (for example, ground up with stone grinders, made into a flour, and cooked) to become edible. Eventually our ancestors began to plant and reap grains. This development is known as the Agricultural Revolution, and it changed the course of history.

In this chapter, I will take you on a quick trip down food history lane. You'll see that, in addition to the Agricultural Revolution, other major dietary shifts have occurred throughout history, and grains have been involved in each one. Taken together, these changes have taken us very far from the food we were meant to eat. Such a dramatic departure from our original diet has set us up for many health problems, which you'll learn about in this and other chapters.

I'll begin by explaining the diet of our distant Stone Age, or Paleolithic, ancestors who lived 15,000 to 40,000 years ago. Although this may not seem relevant to you and your diet today, it is. By understanding the past, you will get a better sense of what type of diet humans are genetically best suited for—a diet based on simple, whole foods directly off the vine or off the hoof, not a diet based on relatively new foods, such as grains.

If your religious beliefs don't concur with the idea of evolution, consider that however you look at it, the first foods of humans were not grains. Humans are far better adapted to fruits and vegetables as carbohydrate sources than to grains.

From No Grains to a Lot of Grains

Our earliest ancestors were hunter-gatherers. They hunted animals, caught fish and shellfish, and gathered plant foods, especially nutrient-rich, fiber-rich vegetables and small amounts of other foods, such as berries and nuts. They didn't consume any of the newfangled foods in our modern diet—pressed oils or fats, alcohol, refined carbohydrates of any kind, or dairy products (other than mother's milk during infancy). They probably ate no grains at all, except in rare instances, and they certainly never ate cultivated grains, legumes, or refined sugars (with the exception of occasional honey, which was very troublesome to obtain!).

The study of Paleolithic nutrition has been an evolving science over the last several decades. The original research presented by R. B. Lee in the 1960s estimated that our Paleolithic ancestors ate almost twice as many plant foods as animal foods—something many archaeologists still agree with today. In the 1980s, S. Boyd Eaton, M.D., of Emory University, took Lee's assumption of a mostly plant-based diet, plus the idea that very lean meat was eaten, and figured that the Paleolithic diet consisted of 34 percent protein, 21 percent fat, and 45 percent carbohydrates from unrefined sources.[1]

A recent reanalysis of Paleolithic nutrition, conducted by a group of scientists, including Eaton and led by Loren Cordain, Ph.D., of Colorado State University in Fort Collins, presents a slightly different picture. This group's research showed that, whenever it was possible, hunter-gatherers consumed more animal food than plant food (say, 65 percent compared to 35 percent). Keep in mind, though, that not all the animal food was protein. To get the maximum amount of energy for the energy expended hunting, hunter-gatherers hunted mostly large game animals that were higher in fat. Humans can only eat so much protein—up to 35 or 40 percent of total calories—without getting sick and taxing the kidneys, so when higher fat game animals weren't available, they turned to leaner meats and ate more carbohydrates. Based on these assumptions, the macronutrient breakdown of hunter-gatherer diets ranged from 19 to 35 percent protein, 28 to 58 percent fat, and 22 to 40 percent carbohydrates from unrefined sources.[2] By contrast, the American diet today contains approximately 15 percent protein, 34 percent fat, 49 percent carbohydrates (mostly from refined grains), and 3 percent alcohol.[3]

Whichever interpretation you prefer, the Paleolithic diet was very different than our modern diet. First, it was higher in protein, significantly higher in vitamins, phytonutrients, and minerals (except sodium), and lower in carbohydrates. The specific amount of fat varied from area to area. The Paleolithic diet may have had a comparable or higher level of fat than the modern diet does, but it had a very different breakdown in the types of fats. Preliminary research suggests that it probably contained more heart-healthy omega-3 fats, monounsaturated fat, and stearic acid, a type of nonatherogenic saturated fat, than the fat in today's domestic grain-fed animals.[4] The high level of saturated fat in domestic animals is unnatural and results from fattening them up on grain.

Carbohydrates in the Paleolithic diet came entirely from unrefined sources, which keep blood sugar levels more steady, rather than the refined grains and sweets of today, which wreak havoc on blood sugar levels. Even if you believe that Paleolithic people ate a mostly plant-based diet (and less fat), the important thing to understand is that their diet contained virtually no grains.

The composition of the Paleolithic diet is important because our hunter-gatherer ancestors by all accounts had much better health than the people who came after them. The archaeological record shows that when people switched to an agricultural lifestyle and a grain-based diet, the general result was a reduction in stature; an increase in bone abnormalities and diseases, dental caries and enamel defects, infectious diseases, and iron-deficiency anemia; and a shorter life span.[5] In addition, the agricultural lifestyle required considerably more work than that of the hunter-gatherers.[6] Just think of planting the grain, harvesting it, separating the chaff from the grain, grinding it with a grindstone, mixing the flour with water, preparing a dough, and cooking the dough. That's quite a lot of work!

Why Did People Adopt a Grain-Based Agriculture?

If an agricultural lifestyle involved more work and resulted in poorer health, why did our ancestors ever decide to adopt it? That question has perplexed scientists for decades.

One possible explanation is a purely practical one. Large animals were gradually becoming extinct at the time because of both climatic changes and overhunting to support increasing numbers of people. Since humans cannot eat only protein, they might have been forced to find an additional source of food—carbohydrates from grains in place of the fat they previously received from large game.[7] Eating grains allowed increasing numbers of humans to survive (but definitely not thrive), especially during the winter months, when few other sources of carbohydrates were available.

Another theory, "the beer and bread hypothesis," comes from a non-nutritional, social, or cultural framework. It took thousands of years for agriculture to spread from the Middle East across Europe, and during that long transition, hunter-gatherer groups and farmers were likely trading. Grains might have been one of the items hunter-gatherers received in trade, but it's unlikely that grains provided a substantial part of their diet. Rather, grains might have been considered rare treats, especially valuable during the winter months when many other wild foods would have been unavailable. If the grains were processed with yeast to make either beer or bread, that would have increased the B vitamin content of the foods, making them more nutritious.[8] In addition, if the grains were processed into beer, that would have made a storable form of grain that had intoxicating properties. Beer would have been something desirable to have for feasts and social occasions, just as it is today, and bread might have been a special occasion food as well. All these factors may have increased the

The Major Dietary Changes Throughout History

The Agricultural Revolution
When: About 10,000 years ago
The Defining Change: The planting and sowing of grains
Health Changes That Occurred As a Result: A reduction in stature; an increase in bone abnormalities and bone diseases; an increase in tooth decay and dental enamel defects; an increase in infectious diseases; an increase in iron-deficiency anemia; a shorter life span

The Industrial Revolution
When: The late 1800s
The Defining Change: The refining of grains and sugar
Health Changes That Occurred As a Result: Nutrient deficiencies; development of degenerative diseases in the masses

The Fast-Food Revolution
When: The mid-1900s to the present
The Defining Change: The combining of refined grains with unhealthy fat, sugar, salt, and/or chemical additives to make convenience foods
Health Changes That Occurred As a Result: Huge increase in obesity and Type 2 diabetes

prestige and social value of grains. High-status people in hunter-gatherer groups might have started to include small amounts of grain-derived food and drink in their diet, then eventually added more grain to their diet, and other people followed.

Yet one more provocative idea is the opioid or exorphin theory proposed in 1993 by Greg Wadley and Angus Martin, researchers at the

The Pluses and Minuses
of the Agricultural Revolution

+ It created a food system that sustained increasing populations around the world and allowed the development of culture, technology, and scientific knowledge.

— It set humans up for diseases and health problems their distant, non-grain-eating ancestors never experienced.

University of Melbourne in Australia.[9] A considerable amount of research indicates that grains and dairy products aren't just food; they also contain opioid substances called exorphins. Researchers have always been very cautious in discussing the possible behavioral effects of exorphins found in normal amounts of grains and dairy products, but the evidence certainly suggests that exorphins have druglike effects and may be, to some degree, addictive. (You'll learn more about exorphins in Chapters 5 and 6.) Wadley and Martin propose that once patches of wild grain appeared, humans learned to process grains to make them more edible, and eating these foods produced a sense of reward or comfort (just like many opioid drugs can cause). Humans then began to favor grains, crave them, and eat more of them—in other words, our early ancestors became hooked on them.

This theory is engaging because many people go crazy over grain-based foods. Virtually all of us have experienced cravings for grain-based foods or the feeling that we can "make room" for more pasta, pizza, or dessert, but can't have another bite of meat or vegetables. Meats and vegetables simply don't have the same opioidlike substances that grain-based foods have. The opioid effect of grains may not be the sole reason for the adoption of agriculture, but it may have been a partial or significant contributor along with other factors.

Whatever the reason for the grain-based Agricultural Revolution, it spread slowly but surely throughout most of the world. The adoption of agriculture is often written about in glorious terms that focus on all the benefits of this new way of living. But the truth is the Agricultural Revolution really brought a mixed bag—both good and bad—as most forms of progress or innovation do. On the plus side, the Agricultural Revolution did create a food system that sustained increasing numbers of people and it enabled humans to create modern culture and technology and to develop and expand scientific and medical knowledge. The negative side, though, is a big one: it set up humans for diseases and health problems their distant, non-grain-eating ancestors never experienced.

Health Problems Associated with the Spread of Agriculture

The expansion of agriculture didn't happen overnight. Grain-based agriculture began with planting and sowing wild species of wheat and barley in the Middle East in approximately 9000 B.C. However, it took 5,000 years to spread through the middle of Europe and reach the fringes of Europe, such as Ireland and Sweden. It is noteworthy that modern Europeans who have the highest frequencies of celiac disease—a severe reaction to gluten found in wheat, barley, and rye—live in the outskirts of Europe, exactly those areas that have been exposed to gluten grains the shortest amount of time! As you'll learn in Chapter 5, celiac disease results in damage to the intestine, malabsorption, and a wide variety of complications such as iron-deficiency anemia, autoimmune diseases, and infertility. The evolutionary history of celiac disease, at least in Europe, is inextricably linked to the spread of gluten-containing, grain-based agriculture, according to Laura Johnson-Kelly, M.A., an anthropologist from Cornell University in Ithaca, New York.[10]

Johnson-Kelly has also pointed out that celiac disease produces a wide range of bone abnormalities including osteoporosis, rickets (soft, thin, bowed bones), gnarled bones from arthritis, dental enamel defects, and other abnormalities involving long bones and cranial bones.[11] These skeletal abnormalities increased as the cultivation of gluten grains spread throughout Europe and continued to increase as grains became more of a staple. By the Middle Ages, when people in Europe relied on grains for the majority of their calories, bone health was generally horrible, with evidence of dietary stress in many, if not most, skeletons. The decline in bone health could have been caused by many factors associated with a high-grain diet (including its high content of mineral-blocking phytate, which you'll learn about in Chapter 4), but widespread celiac disease is one explanation. Some European populations that adopted agriculture relatively late may not have had any gluten-related health complaints for centuries because these people had a low intake of gluten. However, by the Middle Ages, Europeans were pretty much relying on gluten grains for most of their calories, so it's likely that celiac disease was much more widespread. Whether the gluten in wheat or some other factor in grains contributed to the significant decline in bone health, there's no doubt that bones were stronger and healthier when our ancestors ate meat and vegetables than when they ate a lot of gluten grains.

It's worth noting that even after agriculture developed in other parts of the world, the majority of humanity didn't eat gluten-containing grains.[12] In Asia, rice was the cultivated staple, while in Africa, sorghum and millet were, and in the Americas, corn was (except in some of the northern areas of North America). The people in Australia didn't rely on any grains.[13] Today, however, gluten-based foods (mostly wheat products) have been introduced into all these continents. I have little doubt that people with ancestries from these areas are experiencing health problems from eating gluten grains that their ancestors never had.

Gluten grains may be the most problematic of the grains, but a high intake of nongluten grains has caused plenty of health problems around the world, too. For example, corn is a nongluten grain, but it is particularly low in niacin (vitamin B_3) and tryptophan, an amino acid the body can use to make niacin. A high intake of corn, therefore, has been associated with pellagra, a niacin deficiency disease. After European explorers discovered corn in America and brought it back to Europe, corn became the typical peasant's staple in many areas around the Mediterranean from the mid-1700s to the mid-1800s. As a result, pellagra, characterized by the three d's (dementia, diarrhea, and dermatitis), became a chronic disease in these areas.[14] Pellagra also became a serious public health problem in the southern United States at the beginning of the 1900s. Over the next several decades, it resulted in an estimated six million deaths in the United States.[15] Similar epidemics have occurred in areas of India and Africa when corn was eaten as a staple.

These examples provide historical evidence that a high intake of whole grains has caused nutritional problems, which in turn has caused serious health problems. In Chapter 4, you'll learn about other nutrient deficiency diseases associated with a high intake of grains.

The Emergence of Refined Grains

After the Agricultural Revolution, the next major shift in our diet came during the Industrial Revolution in the late 1800s when the steel-roller mill was developed. This innovation made the refining of whole wheat grain and sugarcane a fast and inexpensive process, and as a result, white flour and white sugar became affordable and easily available to the masses. The effects on health from a diet high in whole grains was bad enough, but things got much worse when populations began to eat refined grains.

Refined wheat flour, or white flour, is stripped of nutrients and fiber and is quite high in carbohydrates. As a result, it contributes to nutrient deficiencies, tooth decay, and many degenerative diseases, especially when it's eaten in conjunction with refined sugar, which it often is. Refined sugar is derived from sugarcane, a member of the large Gramineae or grass/grain family, and it also can be derived from sugar beets.

Refined Grains and Physical Degeneration: Weston Price's Studies

The first researcher to gather an impressive amount of evidence implicating white flour and white sugar in physical degeneration was Weston Price. Price was trained as a dentist in 1893. When he began his practice, he realized that more and more children in the United States were developing tooth decay and other dental problems that their parents had not experienced. He suspected that nutritional changes in the modern diet were responsible, and he ended up doing a truly remarkable thing: he traveled around the world throughout the 1930s, gathering data on the diet and health of more than a dozen nonindustrialized societies from the Arctic to the tropics.

Price found that native people ate different types of whole foods from area to area, but all groups were basically free of chronic disease. In most societies that Price studied, fish, meat, and vegetables formed the bulk of the diet, and grains played little or no role. However, whole grains were important foods for a fraction of the societies Price studied, and a few other societies relied on other high-carbohydrate foods, such as sweet potatoes. Price observed that groups that relied more on grains or tubers as staples generally avoided degenerative diseases, but they tended to have more tooth decay and be less physically developed and less strong than groups that ate more animal foods.

Whatever their traditional diet, natives who became exposed to "white man's foods" and included these foods in their diets had their health decline quickly. Among the health problems that developed were widespread tooth decay; infertility, miscarriages, difficult labor, and birth defects; changes in the shape of the dental arches, head, and face; increased susceptibility to infectious diseases; and more cases of cancer, arthritis, and other chronic diseases.

The Rule of 20 Years

Another astute researcher, Dr. Thomas L. Cleave, traced the development of heart disease, hypertension, diabetes, gallbladder disease, and colitis to the increased intake of refined carbohydrates. In every case Cleave studied, he found that primitive cultures were almost entirely free of these diseases until about twenty years after white flour and white sugar were introduced. This pattern was so consistent that Cleave named the phenomenon the "Rule of 20 Years." Although societies around the world did not exhibit immediate health problems from eating white flour and white sugar, they did slowly but surely develop them over time—just enough time to prevent people from readily connecting the cause with the effect.

This same general pattern also occurred in modern societies. Before the Industrial Revolution, only royalty and the rich ate nutrient- and fiber-stripped white flour because it was labor intensive and costly to produce. Wealthy people consequently became obese and developed degenerative diseases, such as heart disease and adult-onset diabetes, much more often than poor people, who ate whole grains. Once white flour and white sugar became widely available to the general population, insulin-related degenerative diseases—and other conditions brought on by a lack of fiber—started to afflict more and more people. Consider that heart disease was practically unknown in the United States at the beginning of the twentieth century and really began to be a public health problem several decades after wide-scale refining of wheat and sugar began.[16] In a 1943 textbook on heart disease, Paul Dudley White, M.D., President Dwight D. Eisenhower's personal physician during his two heart attacks, explained that when he graduated from medical school in 1911, he had never heard of coronary thrombosis (heart attack). But, by 1943, it was responsible for more than 50 percent of all deaths.[17]

Nutrient Deficiencies Caused by Refined Grains

Even when not in tandem with nutrient-depleting sugar, refined grains all by themselves led to the development of nutrient deficiencies. The most significant example of this involved white or polished rice. In the milling process, rice, like wheat, is stripped of significant percentages of the vitamins and minerals present in the whole grain. Thiamin, or vitamin B_1, is lost to a significant extent (about 75 percent), so in areas where white or polished rice was eaten as an almost exclusive staple, the vitamin B_1-deficiency disease, beriberi, became prevalent. Characterized by general debility, inflammation of nerves, paralysis, and cardiovascular symptoms such as tachycardia, beriberi is a painful disease that can be deadly. In Japan, in the mid-1920s, beriberi resulted in tens of thousands of deaths annually.[18]

The milling of wheat to produce white flour is a nutritional error comparable to that of milling rice. The main difference is that, because Americans have not used white flour as an almost exclusive article in their diet, health problems haven't been as obvious as the more overt problems experienced in parts of Asia.[19] In the 1930s, health professionals did find that many Americans had developed deficiencies of vitamins B_1, B_2, B_3, and iron from eating white bread. A nutritional debate over enriching white flour versus using whole wheat flour ensued. Although animal studies found that white bread enriched with nutrients was nutritionally inferior to whole wheat bread, an American Medical Association nutrition council sided with commercial bread manufacturers and made the decision to require that white flour be enriched with four nutrients, ignoring the fact that more than twenty others are stripped away in the refining process.

Just a few years ago, the government finally acted on twenty-year-old research showing that folic acid protected against the development of neural tube birth defects: it mandated that supplemental folic acid be included in the enrichment process. But numerous other nutrients important for protection against diseases are still missing. Among the most notable are other B vitamins, including vitamin B_6, which is needed for prevention of a key risk factor for heart disease, and chromium, zinc, and magnesium, which protect against Syndrome X and Type 2 diabetes. Although it's misleading, every time you see the word *enriched*, you really should think "deficient." While enriched grains and flours are better than nonenriched, refined grains and flours, they're not as nutritious as whole-grain foods. Whole-grain foods in turn aren't as nutritious as meat and lots of vegetables, which formed the base of our ancestral diet.

The Rise of Grain-Based Convenience Foods

Beginning in the middle of the twentieth century, a faster pace of life—and more and more cars on the road—spurred the development of fast food in restaurants and supermarkets. Once again, grain-based foods were integrally involved in this major diet shift.

The Fast-Food Movement

Between the late 1940s and early 1960s, McDonald's, Carl's Jr., Dunkin' Donuts, Taco Bell, and Domino's Pizza all sprang up. What did these eating places have in common? Food that can be eaten out of hand instead of with a fork, knife, or spoon—in other words, food that was breaded, wrapped in bread, or made with refined grains in some way that made the food convenient and transportable.

Americans loved receiving almost-instant food upon ordering, and fast-food mania swept across the nation over the next several decades. More and more people began eating at fast-food restaurants not only because of convenience but also because they became hooked on the taste. The fast-food industry catered to Americans' taste buds, adding sugar, salt, and fat to everything, which covered up the uninspiring taste of white-flour products. Chemical additives also were added—sometimes to make foods uniform, sometimes to extend their shelf life, and always to benefit manufacturing and not the health of the consumer. As Americans began gobbling up grain-based convenience foods, they unknowingly consumed a lot of other unhealthy ingredients in the process, which added to the disease-causing effects of white-flour products.

Soft drinks were promoted in conjunction with fast-food entrées—just think of "buy a big burger, get a large cola free." So, consumption of soft drinks increased right along with consumption of fast food. Although most people don't realize it, soft drinks are made from grains. Originally sweetened with sugar (which is often from sugarcane, a distant relative of wheat), soft drinks in more recent years have been sweetened with high-fructose corn syrup, which is derived from corn. A high intake of fructose raises blood cholesterol and triglyceride levels, increases free radical production, makes blood cells more prone to clotting, raises insulin levels, and promotes the development of insulin resistance—all factors involved in the development of cardiovascular disease. In other words, chugging all those supersize soft drinks is just one more way in which highly refined grain products contribute to heart disease. Combining soft drinks with food mixtures of highly refined grains, highly refined fats, sugar, salt, and chemical additives creates even more serious nutritional problems, and this is where we are today. About a quarter of the American population eats fast food every day.[20]

The Change in Supermarkets

The movement toward easy-to-grab, grain-based convenience foods didn't just occur in restaurants, of course. The same trend occurred in supermarkets and, later, in convenience markets. By polishing rice and degerminating and bleaching flour (and often adding chemical additives), food manufacturers began to realize that they could make grain products so nutritionally sterile that insects wouldn't bother infesting them. The food products would not go bad quickly, if at all, so refined, grain-based convenience products with long shelf lives began making up most of the thousands of items in the inner aisles of grocery stores. Consumers thought they were getting variety, but they really weren't; they were simply buying and eating refined-grain products in many disguised shapes and forms. In addition, since refined-grain convenience foods were so cheap to make, manufacturers and supermarkets heavily promoted them. Coupons were a main promotional tool used, prompting consumers to think they were getting a deal and to buy more. Buying refined-grain products became so much a part of the American lifestyle that most people today can't imagine a diet without them.

Grain products even found their way into the meat purchased in supermarkets and restaurants. Before World War II, more than 90 percent of American cattle was grass fed, not grain fed.[21] That changed because of American grain surpluses, largely caused by government price supports, and because grain fattens cattle more rapidly than grass. During the 1970s, feedlots became commonplace throughout the U.S. farm belt, and grain-fed livestock became a standard not just in the beef industry, but in the production of virtually every other type of meat.

Dietary Changes from the 1970s to the Present

During the 1970s, government and health officials blamed the rise in heart disease on the saturated fat in meat: they never made the connection that too many grains—both in our diets and in the diets of the animals we were eating—were the real problem. Health officials advocated more polyunsaturated fats in place of saturated fats and consumers heeded their advice by adding fats such as corn oil and corn oil margarine—more highly refined grain products! Corn is quite high in omega-6 fatty acids, a type of fat that, in excess, promotes insulin resistance, the underpinning of abdominal obesity, Syndrome X, and Type 2 diabetes. So this advice ended up worsening the health of the nation.

In the 1980s, the fat-free movement became the rage. People responded to the faulty "fat is bad" message by reducing or eliminating meat and loading up on fat-free, usually sugar-rich, refined-grain products, such as fat-free cookies, crackers, and rice cakes. This type of diet is

---

Unhealthy Grain-Based Foods
Through the Decades

The 1970s

Americans began eating more corn oil and corn oil margarine.

The 1980s

Americans began eating more fat-free sweets and snack foods, such as fat-free cookies, crackers, popcorn, and pretzels.

The 1970s–1990s

Americans increased their intake of grain-based foods with a hidden high-fat content, such as cheese pizza, pasta with cheese, Mexican food, and tortilla chips.

The 1990s

Americans began unknowingly eating genetically engineered corn products.

---

a recipe for obesity and Type 2 diabetes. Consequently, the incidence of these conditions skyrocketed out of control in the 1980s and 1990s.

Today we're not quite so fat phobic as then, but that's not necessarily a good thing: we're eating more high-fat, grain-based food combinations (pizza, nachos, quesadillas, pasta with cheese)—combinations that pack on the pounds easily. Sixty-one percent of the American population is now overweight, and this prevalence of obesity is only expected to get much worse, greatly increasing the risk of the big killers in our society: heart disease, Type 2 diabetes, and cancer.

The latest disastrous movement away from our original diet—genetic engineering—has already started. In genetic engineering, genes from one living thing—say, a bacteria, virus, insect, fish, or plant—are implanted into another living thing, thereby creating newfangled foods with built-in pesticides, antinutrients, or other characteristics. Any way you look at it, this dramatic departure from the natural foods we evolved eating is certain to lead to more food allergies, chemical sensitivities, and other health problems (see Chapter 6).

The further we have moved away from the diet we were designed for, the worse it has been for our health. Humans have been putting the wrong fuel in the tank for a long time now and our bodies have been trying to tell us that loudly and clearly.

In the next several chapters, I will give you a more detailed understanding of the little-known problems with grains and how different types of grains are associated with various types of health problems. Chapter 3 starts the discussion by covering refined grains and how they contribute to the development of the most common health problems experienced today.

CHAPTER 3

The Trouble with Refined Grains

Refined grain products are the rule in the North American diet. They come in lots of different forms: pastas, rolls, breads, muffins, cookies, cakes, breakfast bars, cereals, bagels, pretzels, tortillas, and pizza dough.

Unlike whole grains, which are virtually never eaten and are rarely available in restaurants, refined grains are ubiquitous in our society, found in the fanciest restaurants and the greasiest fast-food places. Consequently, refined grains are difficult to avoid unless you're consciously working at it. Furthermore, no one bothers to think twice about whether refined grains are good foods to include in the diet. Instead, eating refined grains is simply an accepted part of being an American, something everyone is socialized to do.

And herein lies the problem: refined grain products are unhealthy foods. Of course, they don't cause health problems overnight, but they're stripped of blood-sugar-regulating fiber and countless nutrients needed for health. Over time—as Weston Price and Thomas Cleave found out—they subtly and sneakily contribute to serious health problems, especially in the forms and amounts most people eat.

The main refined grain in the diet is white flour, used to make bread, pasta, snack foods, and most desserts. Other refined products from the grain/grass family are fructose and sugar, sweeteners that are often combined with white flour in a variety of products, and white rice, which generally plays a less significant role in our diet than white flour.

The Quality and Quantity of Carbohydrates in Refined Grains

When sizing up the nutritional value of carbohydrates, there are three important things to look at: their glycemic rating, their carbohydrate density, and their nutrient density. When refined grains are put to these tests, they rate poorly across the board.

The Glycemic Rating of Refined Grain Products

The glycemic index is a rating system developed to measure food's effects on blood sugar levels. Refined-grain products, such as bread, breakfast cereals, quick-cooking grains, cookies, corn chips, and pretzels, have a more complex physical structure than simple sugars, so it was always assumed that they would be digested more slowly and would release glucose into the bloodstream more slowly. But when researchers began investigating the glycemic index in the 1980s, they found that most refined grain products act more like simple sugars in the body: they are broken down into blood sugar quickly after being eaten. In other words, they have high glycemic ratings. By contrast, most vegetables (except for potatoes and a few other root vegetables), most fruits (except dried fruits and tropical fruits), dairy products, a few whole grains, and beans have low to moderate glycemic ratings—in other words, they induce more favorable, low to moderate rises in blood sugar.

Is there anything wrong with eating foods that elevate blood sugar? In a word, yes. As my coauthors and I explained in *Syndrome X: The Complete Nutritional Program to Prevent and Reverse Insulin Resistance*, elevated glucose generates hazardous molecules called free radicals in the body, which accelerate aging. Also, excess glucose reacts with and damages proteins in the body, which also ages tissues.

Recent research into the glycemic index has also led to other interesting discoveries. Diets based on low-glycemic carbohydrates improve insulin sensitivity (blood sugar metabolism), blood triglyceride levels, total cholesterol levels, and the ratio of "bad" LDL to "good" HDL cholesterol levels.[1,2,3,4] They also reduce hunger.[5] In one 1999 study, obese teenage boys ate 81 percent more calories after eating two high-glycemic meals of instant oatmeal than after eating two low-glycemic meals of vegetable omelets and fruit.[6] Generally speaking, avoiding high-glycemic foods, such as refined grains, is health promoting, especially for those with blood sugar problems, high cholesterol or triglyceride levels, or problems with being overweight or overeating.

But as helpful as the glycemic index is for understanding an individual food's effects on blood sugar levels, it doesn't give the whole story about how healthy different carbohydrates are for us. For example, fructose—a sweetener often thought of as fruit sugar but really made commercially from corn—ranks low on the glycemic index. Many people, therefore, think fructose is a healthy alternative to common table sugar and a safe sweetener for diabetics. However, this is a big mistake. Fructose doesn't raise blood sugar much, but it does a lot of other bad things: it raises levels of cholesterol and triglycerides; promotes insulin resistance, the condition that is at the core of Type 2 diabetes; and combines with proteins, just like glucose does, to form sticky end-products that damage and age our tissues.

In addition, the glycemic index of a food is determined after subjects eat a certain amount of carbohydrates from a given food. With this type of test, carrots—a very nutritious food—rank high on the glycemic index. Therefore, carrots, you would think, should be avoided. But focusing on the glycemic index alone will lead you astray. Eating a pound of carrots will cause spikes in blood sugar levels, but eating a carrot or two in a mixed meal, as most people generally do, will not significantly raise blood sugar levels. All by itself, the glycemic index is overrated. To get an accurate picture of how healthful various types of carbohydrates are, you also need to take into account the total amount of carbohydrates different foods supply.

The Carbohydrate Density of Refined Grain Products

The carbohydrate density of a food is determined by the amount of digestible carbohydrates—the total grams of carbohydrate in the food minus the grams of fiber (a type of carbohydrate that does not raise glucose levels). The glycemic index and the carbohydrate density of foods are closely aligned in many respects. Foods that have low glycemic ratings, such as nonstarchy vegetables, are low in carbohydrates. Foods that have high glycemic ratings—such as cake, soft drinks, bagels, doughnuts, granola bars, English muffins, and hamburger buns—tend to be high in carbohydrates. However, this isn't always true.

One of America's favorite foods, pasta, is a good case to illustrate this point. Most types of pasta (as long as they are not overcooked) have moderate to low glycemic ratings. This has prompted some health professionals in recent years to advocate eating pasta. However, this advice is ill conceived because pasta is very high in carbohydrates (and calories). One cup of cooked enriched spaghetti has a carbohydrate density of 40 grams of digestible carbohydrates. This is calculated from the total carbohydrate content of a cup of spaghetti, 42 grams of carbohydrates, minus 2 grams of those carbohydrates as fiber. Most people, of course, don't limit themselves to one cup of spaghetti. They often have two, three, four, or five cups of pasta, or more—the "never-ending pasta bowl" syndrome. Common sense alone will tell you that you can't eat large amounts of low-glycemic, but carbohydrate-dense grains without the body having to store away all those extra carbohydrates in the form of fat.

Enter insulin, the hormone that lowers blood sugar levels and promotes the storage of excess fat in the body. If we keep eating carbohydrates that raise glucose levels, the body will keep pumping out lots of insulin to lower blood sugar levels. Just like high glucose levels, high insulin levels are detrimental to health: they promote the storage of fat, increase the risk of several types of cancer (which you'll learn about later in this chapter), and lead in time to the development of insulin resistance—a prediabetic condition in which body cells respond sluggishly to insulin and, therefore, don't process blood sugar efficiently. Insulin resistance can then lead to Syndrome X—a combination of abdominal obesity, high

Sizing Up the Nutritional Value of Refined Grains and Other Carbohydrates

There are three main ways to evaluate the nutritional value of carbohydrates:

- Their glycemic index (how high a food raises blood glucose levels)

- Their carbohydrate density (the total content of digestible carbohydrates)

- Their nutrient density (the nutrients a food provides relative to the amount of calories or carbohydrates it provides)

As you can see, refined grain products rate poorly in all three ways.

Glycemic Index

High glycemic (undesirable)	Low glycemic
Most refined grain products	Nonstarchy vegetables
Sugar and most other sweeteners	Most fruits

Carbohydrate Density

High in carbohydrates (undesirable)	Low in carbohydrates
Refined grain products	Nonstarchy vegetables
Sugar, soft drinks, and fruit juices	Some fruits

Nutrient Density

Low in nutrients (undesirable)	High in nutrients
Refined grain products	Nonstarchy vegetables
Sugar, sweeteners, and soft drinks	Fruits

triglycerides, high cholesterol, and high blood pressure, which greatly increases the risk of heart disease, Type 2 diabetes, and other degenerative diseases and causes us to age faster than we should. So, it's not enough to focus simply on foods that are low or moderate on the glycemic index.

The body's glucose and insulin responses are equally important, and they are influenced by both the amount of carbohydrates and the food's glycemic index.[7,8]

When you evaluate sources of carbohydrates by both their glycemic index and carbohydrate density, refined-grain products rate worse than just about any other type of food. By contrast, nonstarchy vegetables, such as salad greens, asparagus, green beans, and broccoli, come way out on top. The value of vegetables over refined-grain products becomes even more apparent when you also consider their nutrient density, which we'll do shortly.

Based on what is known right now, evaluating carbohydrates according to their carbohydrate density and their glycemic ratings is the best way to select foods that support healthy blood sugar and insulin levels for the public at large. But keep in mind that individuals vary in their glucose and insulin responses to foods. Several nutrition colleagues of mine who specialize in treating delayed food allergies have observed that many hypoglycemics and Type 2 diabetics have had their conditions dramatically improve after identifying and eliminating hidden food allergens—often grains such as wheat—from their diet. One study found that partially digested, druglike substances in wheat gluten did not significantly affect glucose levels but did raise insulin levels.[9] So, if you eat low-glycemic pasta but are sensitive to it, substances in it may have druglike effects or may influence the hormonal system in some way to throw off normal insulin regulation. Research will continue in the area of our individual responses to foods for quite some time, but if you have health problems associated with imbalanced blood sugar or insulin levels and can't figure out why, suspect wheat and other foods that you could be reacting to adversely.

Nutrient Deficiencies and Imbalances in Refined Grains

Most people don't realize it, but refined grains are nutrient-impoverished foods. The process of refining wheat and removing the starchy endosperm away from the bran and germ strips away the following portions of the vitamins and minerals essential for health:[10]

60 percent of the calcium

85 percent of the magnesium

77 percent of the potassium

78 percent of the zinc

68 percent of the copper

76 percent of the iron

86 percent of the manganese

40 percent of the chromium

48 percent of the molybdenum

As you learned in the last chapter, nutrient deficiencies became public health problems in the 1920s and 1930s in the Far East and United States where refined grain products were regularly consumed. This prompted the U.S. government to enact the Enrichment Act of 1942—proof positive that refined grains do not provide the nutrients we need. However, the Enrichment Act didn't go far enough: even today, supplemental amounts of only four vitamins (vitamins B_1, B_2, B_3, and folic acid) and one mineral, iron, are added to refined grain products. Other nutrients are still missing. Some of these nutrients, such as chromium, magnesium, and zinc, are needed to help the body properly use grains and other carbohydrates for fuel. Other nutrients, such as potassium and calcium, are needed to perform other vital functions, such as relaxing muscles and building bones. Eating a lot of white-flour products that don't provide many of these nutrients, therefore, can lead to subtle, preclinical nutrient deficiencies over time. The more refined grain and sugary foods we eat, the less we eat nutritious foods that provide the nutrients missing from refined grains; and the more likely we are to develop suboptimal intakes or outright nutrient deficiencies that prevent our bodies from functioning at their best.

Keep in mind, also, that refined grains, like the whole grains they're derived from, contain no vitamin B_{12} and none of the important antioxidants—vitamin C, vitamin A, and beta-carotene. (The only exception to this rule is yellow corn, which does contain some beta-carotene.) If refined grains form a major part of the diet and crowd out other foods, such as meats, fruits, and vegetables, which supply these nutrients, deficiencies of these vitamins also can become problems.

About the only good thing you can say about the refining process is that it also strips away some of the antinutrients found in whole grains, and therefore probably makes the grains a little more digestible. (You'll learn more about the antinutrients in grains in the next chapter.) However, even if you seem to tolerate refined grains better than whole grains, don't for a moment fool yourself into thinking refined grains are better for you. Refined grains provide a lot of carbohydrates (and calories), very little fiber, and few nutrients. Whole grains provide a lot of carbohydrates (and calories), some more fiber and nutrients, but also some more antinutrients. In terms of nutritional value per calories, neither one comes close to the value of nonstarchy vegetables, which are low in carbohydrates and chock-full of blood-sugar-balancing fiber, antioxidants, and other nutrients needed for health.

Heather's Story

Heather, a twenty-two-year-old college student, came to see me because she wanted to lose weight. She was a typical college student, immersed in both her studies and social fun and always on the run. On an average day, Heather ate a bagel or croissant on the go for breakfast, a muffin for a midmorning snack, a burrito or sandwich and soft drink for lunch, cookies for a late afternoon pick-me-up, pizza and cola or beer for dinner, and pretzels or popcorn at bars and the movies. Her main complaint was that she was about twenty pounds overweight and couldn't fit into her favorite clothes. However, when I questioned Heather a bit further, I also found out that she was often bloated, didn't have as much energy as she wanted, sometimes had trouble concentrating on her studies, and suffered from premenstrual irritability and mood swings.

After looking over her food diary, I explained to Heather that she was eating a lot of junk food with calories but few nutrients—just a slight step up from eating sugar (nothing but empty calories) all day long. She needed to eat real food and replace all or most of those grain products with a lot more vegetables and protein. This was standard advice for me to give, but Heather was totally shocked by what I said. I got the impression she thought I was radical. At the end of our session, Heather thanked me for my advice, but I wasn't sure I would hear from her again.

Six months or so later, Heather called me. She said that she "was blown away" by my nutritional advice, and she needed some time for the information to sink in. To prove to herself that the advice I gave her was off base, Heather surfed the Internet and did some research into the matter. However, to her surprise, she ended up finding more evidence to back up what I said. So, Heather gradually cut down on the many refined-grain products in her diet, and her body began to respond: She lost several pounds and began feeling more energetic and mentally focused.

When the school year ended, she went back to live with her mother for the summer. Her mother, a client of mine, was already following my advice to eat against the grain, so it became a lot easier for Heather to eat that way, too.

Avoiding refined-grain products worked liked a charm. Over the next few months, Heather lost all her excess weight and gained more energy than she ever expected. As an unexpected bonus, her premenstrual symptoms went away as well. Heather called me to say thanks for showing her the secret to better health and easy weight control.

Harmful Ingredients Often Combined with Refined Grains

Nutritionally speaking, refined grains are bad enough all by themselves, but they're often made worse by being combined with unhealthy ingredients to make common convenience foods. Pick up virtually any convenience food, and you'll almost always see one or more of the following ingredients.

Sugar

Sugar is a highly refined product made from either sugarcane or beets. It is most usually found as table sugar or sucrose, but also found in variations such as brown sugar, raw sugar, turbinado sugar, cane juice, cane syrup, and dehydrated cane juice crystals. A high-glycemic, high-carbohydrate food that supplies essentially no nutrients, sugar is a prime contributor to all diseases involving "overconsumptive malnutrition," including excess weight, obesity, heart disease, and Type 2 diabetes. In addition, sugar suppresses immune function, not only reducing the ability of white blood cells to track and attack bacteria but also reducing the production of antibodies, which protect against viruses and other invaders.

When large-scale commercial refining of sugar began in the late 1800s, sugar was used at first for rare treats. In time, treats and soft drinks made from sugar became more common in the diet, and sugar was added as a sweetener, flavor enhancer, or preservative to more and more foods—everything from pizza sauce to crackers. The consumption of sugar in the United States escalated throughout the 1900s to an all-time high of more than one hundred pounds per person per year in the early 1970s. Since that time, sugar consumption has dropped and has been partially replaced by a higher intake of corn-based sweeteners, most notably high-fructose corn syrup.

High-Fructose Corn Syrup

Compared to sugar, high-fructose corn syrup (HFCS) is sweeter and easier to handle during processing, has a longer shelf life, and is cheaper. Consequently, in the 1970s, shortly after HFCS was developed, manufacturers began using more HFCS and less sugar in soft drinks and in grain-based convenience foods and sweets, such as doughnuts, breakfast bars, muffins, and cookies. Today, HFCS has replaced a good portion of the sugar used in food processing. The average American now consumes 83 pounds of corn sweeteners (such as high-fructose corn syrup) per year, 65 pounds of refined sugar per year, and a small amount of other sweeteners. This makes a total of 150 pounds of caloric sweeteners per year, up from 120 pounds in 1970, and much of this is hidden in grain-based foods, ranging from bagels to ready-to-eat breakfast cereals.[11]

The switch to more hidden HFCS in the diet (and more total sweeteners) has made America's health problems even worse than they were before. To explain, sugar is a compound that breaks up into equal parts of glucose and fructose. HFCS, in contrast, is a blend of 55 percent fructose and 45 percent glucose. (As the name implies, HFCS is high in fructose.) Fructose, it turns out, contributes to insulin resistance and heart disease more than glucose does.

Soft Drinks Derived from Refined Grains?

Most people don't realize it, but soft drinks are made with highly refined-grain ingredients. Originally sweetened with sugar (often from sugarcane, a distant relative of wheat), most soft drinks today are made with high-fructose corn syrup, a sweetener made from corn. The fructose in high-fructose corn syrup contributes to insulin resistance and heart disease more than sugar does. In addition, soft drinks provide a lot of calories and no nutrients. So, instead of thinking of soft drinks as thirst quenchers that are an everyday part of life, think of them as what they really are: The most refined grain product that there is and one of the most important to avoid for long-term health and weight control.

The first alarms about the dangers of fructose were sounded by British researcher John Yudkin, M.D., Ph.D., in the late 1960s. In laboratory and human tests, Yudkin found that sugar (sucrose) increased blood pressure and blood levels of cholesterol, triglyceride, uric acid, insulin, and cortisol, which are all associated with an increased risk of heart disease. More surprising, though, was that all these adverse health effects were magnified when Yudkin substituted fructose for sucrose in his experiments.

Eating more fructose in place of sucrose (without even knowing it) is in large part what Americans have been doing over the last few decades. The result has been that conditions associated with insulin resistance—namely, obesity and Type 2 diabetes—have become nationwide epidemics. Consequently, more people than ever are at strong risk for heart disease, the number one cause of death.

Bad Fats (Trans-Fats and Omega-6 Vegetable Oils)

Refined sweeteners aren't the only refined foods added to refined grain products: refined fats are, too. These include: trans-fatty acids, found in partially hydrogenated oil, margarine, vegetable shortening, and oils used in high-temperature, deep-fat frying, and vegetable oils, such as soybean oil, safflower oil, sunflower oil, corn oil, and cottonseed oils, which are high in omega-6 fatty acids.

Just as highly refined grain and sugar products weren't eaten (at least by the masses) before the Industrial Revolution, highly refined fats weren't eaten either. Crisco, a vegetable shortening made out of partially hydrogenated oil and typically used in baking with refined flour, went on sale in 1911. Large-scale, solvent extraction of plants to make commercial vegetable oils followed in the 1930s. In the 1960s and 1970s, government officials advocated the use of omega-6-rich oils and vegetable shortening, and food companies added these oils (especially partially hydrogenated versions) to everything from cookies and bread to frozen breaded entrées and snack foods. These refined fats are hidden in a wide range of refined-grain products today.

The increased use of refined fats in the United States contributed to more serious health problems. Both omega-3 (which is primarily found in fatty fish) and omega-6 fatty acids are essential for health; however, they need to be balanced, in a ratio of between 1:1 and 4:1, for optimal health. Too many omega-6 fatty acids and too few omega-3 fatty acids in the diet promote insulin resistance, obesity, and inflammation in the body.

What does this have to do with refined grains? Although they're low in fat, grains all by themselves have a high omega-6-to-omega-3 ratio. When grains are combined with vegetable oils such as soybean oil or cottonseed oil in convenience foods, their omega-6-to-omega-3 imbalance and their fat content are made worse.

Trans-fats, which are even more common in processed foods, also promote obesity, insulin resistance, and Syndrome X. What's more, they double the risk of heart disease. So, when grains are combined with partially hydrogenated oils in countless convenience foods that many North Americans eat every day, it's understandable why heart disease continues to be the nation's number one health problem—and why obesity and Type 2 diabetes, which greatly increase the risk of heart disease, are developing earlier and earlier in life.

Food Additives

Food additives—substances that are added to food but aren't food—are combined with refined-grain products for a number of manufacturing reasons. Supposedly safe, many of them pose real or potential dangers to our health.

There are a number of reasons to be concerned about food additives. First, the Food and Drug Administration (FDA) has relaxed safety standards and allowed small amounts of carcinogenic (cancer-causing) substances to be used in food, according to Christine Hoza Farlow, D.C., author of *Food Additives: A Shopper's Guide to What's Safe and What's Not* (Escondido, Calif.; KISS for Health Publishing, 1999). Second, many food additives that aren't carcinogenic cause other harmful effects, such as kidney problems, heart trouble, or serious allergic reactions. Third, some additives in common use now, and considered to be safe, will probably one day be banned.

Perhaps the most compelling reason to be concerned is that there are more than three thousand approved food additives, but nobody has ever tested them in combination with each other. Most packaged, refined-grain products contain a variety of additives, not just one. By combining several different additives, the harmful effects are likely magnified.

The following are a few examples of common food additives you might find in refined-grain convenience foods.

- Artificial colors, labeled as "artificial color," "U.S. certified food color," or "FD&C," followed by a color and number (such as "FD&C Citrus Red No. 2"). They are often used in candies, cereals, and soft drinks made to appeal to kids. Some artificial colors contribute to hyperactivity in children; some may contribute to learning and visual disorders or nerve damage; and others are carcinogenic.

- Preservatives BHA and BHT, common ingredients in some cereals. Experiments have found that BHA and BHT can cause behavioral problems, birth defects, and cancer.

- Monosodium glutamate (MSG), a flavor enhancer found in Chinese food, frozen TV dinners, snack foods, and other convenience foods.

Ingredient Lists of Some Common Foods

Nabisco Original Wheat Thins: enriched flour (wheat flour, niacin, reduced iron, thiamine mononitrate, riboflavin, folic acid), partially hydrogenated soybean oil, defatted wheat germ, sugar, cornstarch, high-fructose corn syrup, salt, corn syrup, malt syrup, leavening (calcium phosphate, baking soda), vegetable colors (annatto extract, turmeric oleoresin), malted barley flour.

Kellogg's Homestyle Eggo Waffles: enriched wheat flour (wheat flour, niacin, reduced iron, thiamin mononitrate, riboflavin, folic acid), whey, partially hydrogenated soybean oil, eggs, water, leavening (baking soda, sodium aluminum phosphate, monocalcium phosphate), sugar, salt, calcium carbonate, niacinamide, reduced iron, yellow #5, vitamin A palmitate, thiamin hydrochloride, riboflavin, pyridoxine hydrochloride, yellow #6, vitamin B_{12}.

Kraft Stove Top Stuffing Mix (for chicken): enriched wheat flour (wheat flour, niacin, reduced iron, thiamin mononitrate, riboflavin, folic acid), high fructose corn syrup, dried onion, salt, partially hydrogenated soybean and/or cottonseed oils, hydrolyzed soy and corn protein, yeast, cooked chicken and chicken broth, soy flour, celery, maltodextrin, monosodium glutamate, whey, parsley flakes, spices, sugar, onion powder, caramel color, turmeric, disodium inosinate and disodium guanylate, sodium sulfite, BHA, BHT, propyl gallate and citric acid (preservatives).

Nabisco Oreo Cookies: sugar, enriched wheat flour (contains niacin, reduced iron, thiamine mononitrate, riboflavin, folic acid), vegetable shortening (partially hydrogenated soybean oil), cocoa, high fructose corn syrup, corn flour, whey, cornstarch, baking soda, salt, lecithin, vanillin (artificial), chocolate.

MSG is a common cause of allergic reactions and has caused brain damage in animal experiments.

Although few researchers have been able to study and evaluate how far-reaching the effects of food additives are on our health, I believe that hidden food additives in our diet certainly contribute to many health problems North Americans are experiencing and that they should be avoided as much as possible. Common sense alone should cause you to think twice about picking up any food with a long list of unrecognizable, hard-to-pronounce ingredients.

A Combination of Harmful Ingredients

More often than not, the refined-grain products that line supermarket shelves and that are eaten in many restaurants have a combination of two or more of these hazardous, newfangled ingredients with no nutritional value. Many products have all the ingredients, for example: sugar, high-fructose corn syrup, soybean oil, partially hydrogenated oil, and artificial colors. When you consider the disease-promoting effects of all these ingredients together with the disease-promoting effects of refined grain products, it's no wonder why degenerative diseases are common today.

Rob's Story

Rob, a fifty-one-year-old business executive, contacted me at the urging of his wife and daughter. Rob was busy with his work and had little time to worry about his diet. Consequently, his health was paying for it: he had a pot belly, high blood pressure, and high blood triglyceride levels. He also had already had one "mini-heart attack." His wife and daughter were concerned that if he didn't do something soon to improve his health, it would be too late.

I talked with Rob on the phone before setting up a consultation with him and suggested he buy a copy of the book I coauthored, *Syndrome X*. By reading it beforehand, he could learn a lot before meeting with me.

A decisive man with a no-nonsense attitude, Rob read the book quickly and was thrilled by the information—information he had never heard before. He certainly had never been told he had Syndrome X or that he could reverse all his health problems if he changed his diet and took certain supplements. He took this information and ran with it, changing his diet to focus on fish, meat, nuts, and vegetables. Since then, he has never deviated from the program and has even persuaded his regular lunch hangouts to offer tasty, innovative, grain-free fare.

The result? Today, Rob is thirty pounds lighter, has dropped five inches from his waist size, and is off all the medications he had been taking for his various heart disease risk factors. Furthermore, he looks twenty years younger, an unexpected change both he and his wife are thrilled with.

Health Problems Associated with Refined Grains

Eating refined grains produces adverse metabolic consequences similar to those that the body experiences when we eat refined sugars. As mentioned, most refined grain products provoke our blood sugar (or glucose) levels to shoot up, and the body produces insulin to lower glucose levels down to normal levels. Sometimes, in the earlier stages of impaired glucose tolerance, the body produces too much insulin, which causes blood sugar to drop too low, a condition known as reactive hypoglycemia. This is a sure sign the body cannot cope with refined grains and sugars and is headed for more serious glucose tolerance problems in the future.

As years of eating high-glycemic, refined-grain products go on, the body pumps out high levels of insulin to control glucose levels and keep blood sugar in a normal range. Eventually, though, the body becomes overwhelmed by so much insulin and doesn't respond as efficiently to insulin's blood-sugar-lowering effects—a condition known as insulin resistance. (This condition is very much like taking so much of a drug that the drug loses its effectiveness and a person has to take more of the drug to get the same effect.) When insulin resistance occurs, the body compensates by churning out even more insulin to keep glucose levels in check. This combination of insulin resistance and high insulin levels can go on silently for years or decades without the person knowing it, while the excess insulin does damage and sets disease into motion inside the body.

Everything has its breaking point, though, and if the pancreas pumps out high levels of insulin for too long, one of two things will happen: body cells become even less responsive to the action of insulin or the work-horse pancreas eventually poops out and stops producing adequate amounts of insulin. In either case, glucose levels start to creep up, first into prediabetic ranges and then into diabetic ranges.

Therefore, *the two main metabolic consequences of eating a lot of refined grains are: high insulin levels (combined with insulin resistance) and high glucose levels.* Both of these, you'll see, in time lead to degenerative diseases and other forms of ill health.

Health Problems Associated with High Insulin Levels

Insulin is a hormone that has far more fundamental roles in the body than lowering blood sugar. It is a powerful mitogen: it stimulates the division of cells and the activation of genes.[12] Prolonged exposure to high levels of insulin actually accelerates the aging of cells, or makes cells act like older cells. It shouldn't be surprising, therefore, that high insulin levels contribute to most, if not all, diseases of aging.

Cardiovascular Disease, Type 2 Diabetes, and Syndrome X

Let's start with cardiovascular disease and Type 2 diabetes. High insulin levels are a strong, independent risk factor for both diseases. In addition, high insulin levels either directly or indirectly lead to other strong risk factors for cardiovascular disease and Type 2 diabetes, such as upper-body ("apple-shaped" or abdominal) obesity, abnormal blood fat levels (high triglycerides and high cholesterol or poor ratios of high-density lipoprotein to low-density lipoprotein cholesterol), and high blood pressure. This cluster of symptoms is known as Syndrome X or the insulin-resistance syndrome. Each component of Syndrome X increases the risk of heart disease and diabetes, and a combination of two or more of these components has an additive, or cumulative, effect in increasing the risk. Recent research has shown that high levels of C-reactive protein, a marker of chronic, subclinical inflammation, are associated with high insulin

The Many Conditions Associated with Insulin Resistance and High-Insulin Levels

Obesity (especially abdominal obesity)

High blood pressure

High blood cholesterol or poor LDL-to-HDL cholesterol ratios

High blood triglycerides

Syndrome X (all the above conditions or a combination of several)

Cardiovascular disease

Type 2 diabetes

Polycystic ovary syndrome (PCOS)

Cognitive disorders, dementia, and Alzheimer's disease

Liver, pancreatic, endometrial, breast, prostate, and colon cancer

Nearsightedness

Reductions in the age of female puberty

levels and are a part of Syndrome X and Type 2 diabetes.[13,14] Elevated levels of C-reactive protein are another factor that greatly increases the risk of cardiovascular disease.[15,16]

Polycystic Ovary Syndrome (PCOS)

Another disorder associated with insulin resistance and high insulin levels that's related to Syndrome X is polycystic ovary syndrome (PCOS), a condition in which a woman's eggs mature in the ovary but are not released. PCOS is the most common cause of infertility among women in the United States, affecting approximately 6 to 10 percent of women of childbearing age.[17] Common symptoms of PCOS are irregular menstrual periods (usually eight or less per year), cysts that develop in the ovaries, elevated blood levels of male sex hormones such as testosterone, excess facial hair, acne, and often excess weight. Studies have shown that high insulin levels stimulate the production of male sex hormones by the ovaries and may impede ovulation and contribute to infertility. In other words, high levels of insulin affect other hormones, upsetting hormonal balance in the body. Not only does PCOS come with its own health problems, but like Syndrome X, PCOS increases the risk of other serious diseases associated with insulin resistance, such as Type 2 diabetes.

Cognitive Disorders and Some Types of Cancer

High insulin levels are associated with still other diseases of aging. Several studies have established insulin resistance and high insulin levels as factors in cognitive disorders, impaired thinking processes, dementia, and even Alzheimer's disease.[18,19,20] There is also substantial evidence that elevated levels of insulin increase the risk of liver, pancreatic, endometrial, breast, and colorectal cancer. As one example of the refined grain connection to these conditions, consider that a high intake of breads and cereals increases the risk of colorectal cancer by 70 percent.[21] Researchers believe that the high-glycemic load of white flour and sugary foods causes the body to compensate by secreting high levels of insulin, and high insulin, in turn, promotes the growth of colorectal tumors.[22] Consider also that a high intake of refined carbohydrates doubles the risk of Type 2 diabetes, and Type 2 diabetics have an increased risk of developing several cancers, such as colorectal, prostate, breast, and endometrial cancers.

More Insulin Connections

The web of diseases and abnormalities associated with insulin resistance and high insulin levels seems to be far reaching and complex. Researchers will likely be ironing out all the insulin connections to various ailments for decades. The latest connection comes from researcher Loren Cordain, Ph.D. In an article entitled "Syndrome X: Just the Tip of the Hyperinsulinemia Iceberg?," Cordain points out that the high insulin levels that go hand in hand with insulin resistance cause a cascade of hormonal shifts that favor unregulated cell growth in a variety of tissues. This unregulated cell growth may contribute not only to PCOS and breast, prostate, and colon cancers but also to, believe it or not, myopia (nearsightedness), acne, and the longtime trends for increased stature and earlier ages of female puberty (menarche).[23]

Although it seems hard to believe that eating a lot of refined grains sets the stage for such a myriad of health problems, research now shows us that it does. To prevent serious degenerative diseases and minor health aggravations, the healthiest thing you can do both for yourself and your children is to avoid refined grains and sugars that promote elevated insulin levels.

Health Problems Associated with High Glucose Levels

As if the adverse effects on health from high insulin levels weren't bad enough, high glucose levels are partners with high insulin levels in the metabolic crime that refined-grain products precipitate. In the short term, eating refined-grain products can cause huge (but temporary) spikes in blood glucose levels, which the body normalizes by producing a lot of blood-sugar-lowering insulin. In the long term, eating refined-grain products can lead to insulin resistance and high insulin levels, which can increase the liver's production of glucose or lead to the pancreas becoming exhausted—both of which will result in chronically elevated glucose levels. Even slightly high blood glucose levels greatly increase the risk of Type 2 diabetes,[24] and Type 2 diabetes carries with it a greatly increased risk of most of the diseases of aging—coronary heart disease, stroke, blindness, nerve disorders, kidney disease, some types of cancer, and, in men, impotence.

Accelerated Aging

High glucose does its damage in two main ways. First, when glucose is burned in the cells, a lot of energy and a small number of free radicals are produced. Free radicals are destructive molecules that damage cells and

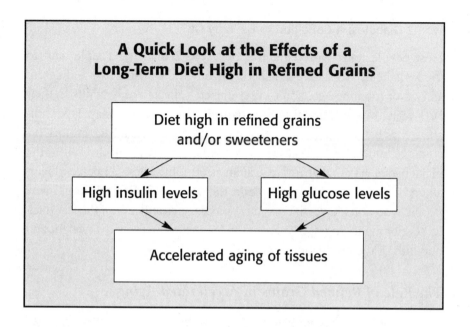

A Quick Look at the Effects of a Long-Term Diet High in Refined Grains

Diet high in refined grains and/or sweeteners

High insulin levels

High glucose levels

Accelerated aging of tissues

age them. The more high-glycemic foods, such as refined grains, are eaten, the more glucose is burned, and the more free radicals are produced. Furthermore, even on its own—without going through the burning process (or Krebs cycle) inside cells—excess glucose in the blood can generate large amounts of free radicals. The more free radicals in the body (without being balanced with antioxidants, protective molecules that neutralize free radicals), the faster cells are damaged and the body ages. Elevated levels of free radicals have also been implicated in the development of virtually every disease. This means that high glucose is likely an exacerbating, if not a causative, factor in a great many diseases.

There's another way high glucose ages the body: it reacts with and damages proteins in organs and tissues, forming *advanced glycation endproducts* (AGEs). AGEs toughen proteins and age cells. Think of wrinkled skin—one good example of the age-accelerating effect of AGEs. Often, the combination of AGEs and free radicals leads to many of the complications of Type 2 diabetes. For example, both free radicals and AGEs damage the eye lens and can cause cataracts. Not surprisingly, diabetics have an above-normal risk of developing cataracts.

Type 2 Diabetes: A Condition to Be Wary Of

Most people don't worry much about Type 2 diabetes. People tend to think diabetes won't happen to them, but the statistics tell a different story. Not too long ago, adult-onset diabetes affected only adults in their later years, but that situation has changed dramatically. Today, Type 2 diabetes has ballooned into an epidemic that now afflicts all age groups, including children as young as ten years old. All throughout the 1990s, the incidence of Type 2 diabetes rose at an astounding rate—33 percent overall and 70 percent among people in their thirties.[25] What's more, many people who don't have diabetes have prediabetes and are on the fast track to developing it. Today, 61 percent of Americans are now overweight and one-fifth of the population is obese.[26]

The Role of Refined Grains in Accelerated Aging

The key points to remember are: Aging is the accumulation of damaged cells, and Type 2 diabetes is a classic example of accelerated aging throughout the body. Both high glucose levels and high insulin levels speed up the aging process, so avoiding foods that provoke high glucose and insulin, such as refined-grain products and concentrated sweeteners, is one of the most important things you can do to promote health and stave off disease.

You might think that you should replace harmful refined grains with whole grains. However, contrary to what you might have heard, eating a lot of whole grains isn't the best dietary solution for countering the problems with refined grains. Whole grains aren't quite as bad for blood sugar levels as refined grains, but they have plenty of other nutritional problems, which contribute to other types of health problems, such as nutrient deficiencies and autoimmune diseases. You'll learn about those problems next.

CHAPTER 4

The Trouble with Whole Grains

Many nutritionists recommend whole grains in place of refined grains, and at first thought this sounds like good dietary advice. On paper at least, whole grains contain more nutrients. They also have more blood-sugar-regulating fiber. Because of that fiber, they generally rank lower on the glycemic index and offer more protection against Type 2 diabetes and heart disease than refined grains.[1,2]

However, whole grains have numerous nutritional shortcomings that make these foods far less beneficial to health than they've been made out to be. Their key nutritional downfalls include a high carbohydrate content, antinutrients that impair the absorption of minerals such as calcium, iron, and zinc, and lectins that wreak havoc with intestinal and immune function. The more that whole grains are eaten, the more their nutritional shortcomings aggravate body function and lead to serious health problems. Ironically, many people switch from a high refined-grain diet to a high whole-grain diet in a search for better health but actually set themselves up for conditions such as bone problems, iron-deficiency anemia, and autoimmune conditions.

The Quality and Quantity of Carbohydrates in Whole Grains

In the last chapter, I explained that there are three main ways to classify carbohydrates. Each system of classification helps highlight the pros and cons of various types of carbohydrates. When evaluated in these three ways, whole grains as a group are better in many ways than refined grains but paradoxically worse in some of the ways that people usually consider them better.

The Glycemic Rating of Whole Grains

As a general rule, whole grains rank lower on the glycemic index—that is, they cause lower blood sugar responses—than refined grains. This is largely because of the fiber they contain, which slows the digestion and absorption of glucose into the bloodstream. As the fiber goes up in a food, the glycemic index comes down.

But fiber isn't the only component that influences the body's glucose response to a food. Particle size has an important influence, too. The more grains are processed—that is, the more grains are ground down into finer and finer forms—the more these foods tend to raise blood sugar. A few cases in point:

- Instant oatmeal has a higher glycemic rating (or raises glucose higher) than old-fashioned, regular-cooking oatmeal.
- Rice cakes have a much higher glycemic rating than brown rice.
- Rye or wheat crackers have higher glycemic ratings than cooked rye or wheat grains.
- Cream of rye or wheat cereals have higher glycemic ratings than cooked rye or wheat kernels.

While whole-grain foods in their less processed forms tend to be better for blood sugar control, many whole-grain foods that people think are wholesome wreak havoc with blood sugar balance. Take whole wheat bread, for example. Based on my initial consultations with clients, if people are going to eat any whole-grain food at all, it is usually whole wheat bread. But many types of whole wheat bread have a high glycemic rating, similar to nutrient-deficient white bread! So, switching from white bread to whole wheat bread doesn't do a person much good in promoting lower blood sugar levels. (Switching to eight-grain bread would be slightly better, though.) Eating whole-grain foods may offer a bit more nutritional value than refined-flour products, but it is never as effective a strategy to promote better blood sugar balance as eating nonstarchy vegetables.

The Carbohydrate Density of Whole Grains

As you learned in the last chapter, the body's blood glucose and insulin responses tend to be closely related, but they aren't always totally in sync. The glycemic index in some ways represents the quality of a carbohydrate but it does not take into account the quantity. Quantity is important because, generally speaking, the more that carbohydrate intake is increased, the more insulin the body will produce. Even if a food does not elevate blood sugar very high, it can cause rises in blood insulin levels, which then can aggravate insulin-related conditions such as abdominal obesity, Syndrome X, and heart disease.

Let's consider pasta again. Whole wheat spaghetti has a slightly lower glycemic rating than regular white spaghetti, and it's also slightly lower in carbohydrates. One cup of whole wheat spaghetti has a carbohydrate density of 32 grams of digestible carbohydrates (a total carbohydrate content of 37 grams minus 5 grams of fiber), compared to 38 grams of carbohydrate per cup for regular white spaghetti. So, whole wheat spaghetti is slightly better, but in the grand scheme of things, the difference in 6 grams of carbohydrates isn't very much.

Make no mistake about it, whether whole grain or refined, grain products are very carbohydrate-dense foods. Compared with nonstarchy vegetables on a per-cup or per-serving basis, whole-grain foods have four to forty times more carbohydrates! This means that whole-grain foods— whether they're low glycemic or not—can lead to weight gain and insulin-related health problems if portion sizes and amounts aren't carefully controlled. While whole grains have some attributes over refined

Why Have We Heard Whole Grains Are So Good for Us?

Many people believe that "whole grains protect against disease." This idea is partially true but misleading. Consider that:

- Whole grains generally have more fiber than refined grains, stimulate lower glucose responses, and protect more against heart disease and Type 2 diabetes. However, whole grains aren't as low in carbohydrates (and calories) and as rich in nutrients as nonstarchy vegetables. Whole grains, therefore, are better for us than refined grains, but not as healthful as vegetables.

- People who eat a lot of whole grains are usually healthier than people who eat a lot of refined grains. But whole-grain eaters tend to lead overall healthier lives—they exercise more, tend not to smoke, don't drink as much alcohol, and eat more health-protective fruits and vegetables. Researchers haven't been able to determine that eating whole grains maintains good health without these other factors.

- Whole-grain products do not contain as many harmful, newfangled ingredients (such as sugar, high-fructose corn syrup, trans-fats, and food additives) as refined-grain products. Fresh vegetables and fruits, though, don't contain any of these ingredients.

grains, they're a poor substitute for nonstarchy vegetables in terms of controlling blood sugar and insulin levels.

Cheri's Story

Cheri, a forty-five-year-old bank teller, had a strong family risk for Type 2 diabetes: her mother had it, her father and grandmother who had both passed away had died from diabetes-related health complications, and her older sister had recently developed it. Knowing her family background and the fact that she had gained ten pounds in the past few years, Cheri was concerned and decided to visit a nutritionist. The nutritionist told her to remove refined grains and other high-glycemic foods from her diet and replace them with foods that ranked lower on the glycemic index, such as whole-grain pasta and beans. Cheri did this and at first thought she felt a little better, but after several months, she realized she couldn't budge her excess weight even though she was exercising like crazy.

After a few more months, she not only couldn't lose weight but began gaining weight. She then went to her doctor for her annual physical. The results were very disappointing. Not only were her "good" HDL cholesterol low and her "bad" LDL cholesterol high, her blood sugar levels had crept up into prediabetic levels.

It was at that point that a friend told her about *Syndrome X*, the book I coauthored. She read it over very carefully and began to follow one of the plans in the book, a diet very similar to the Totally Against-the-Grain Diet in this book, which emphasizes nonstarchy vegetables and no grains. With that simple change in her diet, the excess weight she had gained came off easily without her changing her level of physical activity in the slightest. Five months later, she had another physical: her blood sugar reading had dropped to a perfect-normal level and both her HDL and LDL cholesterol levels were considered excellent.

About a year ago, Cheri sent me an e-mail through our Syndrome X Web site to thank me and tell me how much our plan had helped her. "I always believed whole grains were protective against diabetes and had never been told anything to the contrary," she wrote. "I'm so grateful that you helped me find out that they don't hold a candle to veggies!"

The Nutrients and Antinutrients in Whole Grains

When whole grains are analyzed according to their nutrient density, the picture becomes more complicated than it does when looking at their glycemic rating or carbohydrate density. Refined grains are stripped of more than a dozen nutrients found in whole grains, so it's natural to assume that whole grains are much higher in nutrients that the body can use to promote health. But this isn't really the case. Whole grains have more nutrients, but they also have more antinutrients—substances that impair the absorption or utilization of many nutrients. (The process of milling whole grains into refined grains lowers the levels of vitamins and minerals but it also strips away most of the antinutrients.[3]) Whole grains, therefore, aren't as nutrient dense as most people have been led to believe.

Researcher Loren Cordain, Ph.D., has become an expert on the nutritional shortcomings of grains and has gone a long way toward expanding our knowledge of this important information. In the early 1990s, he came across a few studies on the drawbacks of grains, thought they were interesting, and put them in a file. In time, he came across other provocative papers and kept collecting them. This process continued and accelerated for five long years. He finally organized the information and wrote what is considered the magnum opus on grains, a fifty-four-page paper called "Cereal Grains: Humanity's Double-Edged Sword."[4] Much of the information in this chapter is based on Cordain's paper.

The Role of Whole Grains in Health Problems Around the World

A summary of the nutritional problems with grains follows on the next few pages. It's important to understand that when whole-grain foods are eaten in high amounts—say, 70 percent of the total calories in the diet—they cause or contribute to serious health problems. This is evident in many third world societies around the world. For example, deficiencies of iron, vitamin A, and iodine are the three most important nutritional problems in most developing countries[5] and grains have been implicated as key causes or contributors to each condition.

- Iron deficiency is the most common nutrient deficiency worldwide and poor bioavailability of iron from grain-based diets has been demonstrated to be the main cause of the condition.[6] Iron deficiency is characterized by fatigue, weakness, headaches, and pallor, and the more severe form, iron-deficiency anemia, affects 15 percent of the world's population, with the highest prevalence in developing countries. Numerous factors in whole grains appear to inhibit iron absorption, but the primary one is phytate, which will be covered later in this chapter.

- Vitamin A deficiency is the major cause of blindness among children and also results in greater frequency and severity of, and mortality from, virtually all infectious diseases. The high consumption of grains in developing countries plays a major role in this condition.[7] Not only are whole grains (other than yellow corn) devoid of vitamin A, but when they're eaten in large amounts, they crowd out other foods in the diet (such as beta-carotene-rich fruits and vegetables and vitamin A–rich egg yolks, organ meats, and dairy fats) that could prevent this condition.

- Goiter, a thyroid enlargement condition, afflicts about 200 million people around the world, mainly in Africa. Iodine deficiency is largely regarded to be the main cause of goiter, but in some areas where goiter occurs, there is sufficient iodine in the food supply. Millet, a grain staple regularly consumed in African countries, such as Sudan, plays an instrumental role in goiter development. Millet contains goitrogenic substances that interfere with the formation of thyroid hormones and are not counteracted by iodine intake.[8,9,10]

There are even more examples. Zinc deficiency was first identified in the 1960s among adolescent boys in the Middle East who ate a lot of unleavened whole-grain bread. Vitamin B_{12} and vitamin C deficiencies are quite common in areas of India where the diet is based mainly on whole grains and legumes. (Legumes also have many of the same shortcomings as whole grains.) Also, don't forget that pellagra, a niacin- and tryptophan-deficiency disease, occurred in epidemic numbers in the southeastern United States in the early 1900s among people who used corn as their staple food.

All these examples involved outright nutrient deficiencies that developed from high amounts of grains. In most cases, the primary culprit was some type of antinutrient in whole grains. Doesn't it make sense, then, that people in the Western world who eat diets high in whole grains (whether they're vegetarian, macrobiotic, or any other type) can develop the same nutrient deficiencies? Also, severe nutrient deficiencies develop gradually, not overnight. Isn't it likely that moderate amounts of whole grains can contribute to subtle nutrient deficiencies that many people don't even realize they have? This is an area for future research, but I certainly think this is happening more often than people realize.

Thirteen Nutritional
Shortcomings of Whole Grains[11,12]

1. **Whole grains contain no vitamin C,** a chief antioxidant important for immunity, protection against allergies and asthma, skin health, and prevention of cataracts, cardiovascular disease, and cancer.

2. **Whole grains contain no vitamin A and no vitamin A precursor, beta-carotene (except for yellow corn).** Vitamin A is an anti-infection vitamin, important for the health of mucous membranes, including the skin. Beta-carotene reinforces immunity and plays an important role in the prevention of heart disease and cancer.

3. **Whole grains are not good sources of the B vitamins compared to the calories they provide.** Whole grains are often listed as good sources of B vitamins, but most vitamin charts are calculated by weight. When the B vitamin content in equal-calorie servings of foods is compared, whole grains rank poorly. B vitamins as a group are often called the antistress vitamins, and many of them play important roles in the body's production of energy.

4. **Whole grains contain antinutrients (called pyridoxine glucosides) that reduce vitamin B_6 status.** Vitamin B_6 is important for strong immunity, female hormonal balance, psychological well-being, and prevention of elevated homocysteine, a key heart disease risk factor.

5. **Whole grains contain no vitamin B_{12},** a vitamin critical for nerve and brain health, protection against pernicious anemia, and prevention of elevated levels of homocysteine.

6. **Whole grains contain low levels of bioavailable biotin.** In addition, wheat and sorghum also contain antinutrient elements that depress biotin metabolism. Once called vitamin H, biotin is needed for the metabolism of essential fatty acids that are important for skin, hair, and nail health.

7. **Whole grains indirectly alter the metabolism of vitamin D,** which functions as a hormone and is important for bone health and strong immunity.

8. **Whole grains contain low levels of calcium and numerous other factors that contribute to poor calcium metabolism.** The most abundant mineral in the body, calcium is one of the nutrients crucial for bone and dental health.

9. **Whole grains contain numerous elements that reduce iron absorption.** Iron is needed to prevent iron-deficiency anemia and the fatigue that comes with it.

10. **Whole grains contain phytate and other factors that impair zinc absorption.** Zinc is vital for strong immunity, proper development and growth, and reproductive health.

11. **Whole grains are low in protein** and consistently lower in the essential amino acid lysine than animal proteins. Protein is important for maintaining lean body mass, normal body repair, and strong immunity. Lysine has antiviral effects.

12. **Whole grains contain no taurine or carnitine.** Taurine is a conditionally essential amino acid that has antiarrhythmic and other cardiovascular effects. Carnitine is a vitamin-like nutrient crucial for energy metabolism.

13. **Whole grains are very low in fat, but contain a very high omega-6-to-omega-3 ratio.** This is probably not a problem by itself, but when grains are eaten with omega-6-rich oils, such as corn oil or margarines, the omega-6-to-omega-3 ratio increases. A poor omega-6-to-omega-3 ratio promotes insulin resistance and has proinflammatory effects.

Calcium and Bone Metabolism Problems Caused by Whole Grains

Whole grains cause problems with the metabolism of calcium, which plays an important role in bone health. Calcium balance is far more important for the health of the bones than calcium intake, and the acid-base balance of the diet determines calcium balance.[13] All foods, after digestion and absorption, yield either a net acid or net alkaline load. If the total diet is acidic, the kidneys normalize the balance by using pH buffers from the skeleton to counteract the excess acidity and also by excreting the acid. Foods that are acidic after digestion and absorption are grains, dairy products, nuts, meat, and fish. Whole grains are more acidic than refined grains, and hard cheeses are the most acidic foods. The only alkaline foods are fruits and vegetables.[14]

Therefore, a diet with a lot of grains, meats, and dairy products and very few fruits and vegetables (like the typical American diet) has a negative impact on calcium metabolism and bone health. Switching to a diet high in whole grains and meats or to a lacto-ovo-vegetarian diet (high in dairy products, eggs, and whole grains) is just as bad if not worse. A key point to remember is vegetables and fruits always need to be eaten with grains, meats, and other foods for good calcium balance. The more fruits and vegetables that are eaten, the better it is for bone health. However, recent research shows that many vegetarians aren't eating many fruits and vegetables[15]—they're really more "grainarians" than vegetarians—and doing this can deplete calcium in the body and negatively impact bone health just as much as eating the typical American diet.

The acid-base factor is probably the most critical dietary factor influencing bone metabolism, but there are still other ways in which whole grains have a negative influence on calcium status and bone health. Whole grains:

- Are poor sources of calcium
- Have a poor calcium-to-phosphorus ratio, which can negatively impact bone growth
- Have a low calcium-to-magnesium ratio, which tends to decrease calcium absorption
- Have a high content of phytate, which forms insoluble complexes with calcium and makes much of the calcium that is present unavailable for absorption[16]

Whole grains also indirectly alter the metabolism of vitamin D. Vitamin D is an extremely important nutrient for bone health: it is required for calcium to be absorbed and deposited in bone tissue. Deficiency of vitamin D causes rickets in children and a "soft bone" condition known as osteomalacia in adults. Vitamin D deficiency is widespread in populations that eat high levels of unleavened whole-grain breads—and osteomalacia, rickets, and osteoporosis are commonplace in societies where grains provide the major source of calories.[17] The way in which whole grains promote vitamin D deficiency remains unclear, but it's possible that the kidneys don't activate vitamin D into its more active hormone version when there are a lot of grains in the diet.[18]

Given that whole grains have a negative effect on so many nutrients involved in bone metabolism (including zinc, vitamin C, and vitamin B_6), one of the best things you can do to help prevent osteoporosis and other bone problems is to avoid or greatly limit whole grains in your diet and eat a lot more vegetables and fruits.

Phytate in Whole Grains

Phytate has been mentioned briefly already, but it's important to understand this mineral-binding antinutrient in a little more detail. Phytate is not classified as a fiber but is found with insoluble fiber in whole grains and legumes.

More than fifty years ago, researchers found that bread prepared from high-extraction wheat flour impaired calcium retention. When the phytate in the bread was destroyed, retention of calcium improved. Substantial evidence since then has found that phytate combines not only with calcium but also with iron, zinc, and magnesium and significantly blocks their absorption.

The more whole grain and bran a food contains, the more phytate it contains. In other words, the more you eat whole-grain foods, the higher your intake of phytate. This is problematic because research has shown that humans do not adapt to habitual high intakes of phytate. Vegetarians experience as much inhibition of mineral absorption as do nonvegetarians.[19]

Native people apparently learned that there were antinutrients in grains that needed to be reduced. They developed methods of processing grains—such as soaking, malting, scalding, fermenting, germinating, and sourdough baking—which decreased the amount of phytate. Baker's yeast in yeasted breads also reduces phytate but not as well as some of the older methods of preparing grain-based foods.

The Adverse Effects of Phytates on Mineral Metabolism

A high intake of phytate from whole grains and beans can lead to deficiencies of iron, calcium, or zinc.

- Symptoms of *iron deficiency* include chronic fatigue, concave-shaped nails, lightheadedness or dizziness, chronic headaches, and skin pallor.

- *Calcium deficiency* occurs primarily at the expense of the skeleton. However, symptoms that may develop as a result of mild to moderate calcium deficiency are anxiety or irritability, muscular tension, twitching muscles, or leg cramps.

- Common symptoms of *zinc deficiency* include weakened immunity, frequent colds and flus, slow wound healing, altered sense of taste and smell, lack of appetite, delayed sexual maturation, skin problems, and white spots on the fingernails.

The role of phytate in the development of iron deficiency, calcium deficiency, and bone diseases has already been covered, but phytate is also a prime contributor to zinc deficiency. Zinc deficiency was first observed among boys in the Middle East who ate a lot of unleavened whole-grain bread called *tanok*, which is high in phytate. They displayed severely stunted growth and delayed sexual development—so much so that seventeen-year-old boys in the Middle East had the height and genitalia development of six- or seven-year-old boys in the United States. Since then, zinc deficiency has been identified among children of many countries. Sometimes it is more subtle in nature than the overt deficiency seen in the Middle East. However, zinc deficiency throughout the world is quite common, may affect nearly one billion people, and may even be as prevalent as iron-deficiency anemia.[20]

Studies have found that retention of zinc in the body is inversely related to the level of phytate in the diet.[21] In other words, the more phytate is consumed, the less zinc is retained. Also, phytate from whole grains has a worse effect on zinc retention than phytate from beans.[22] However, when you eat whole grains combined with beans, that's double trouble for zinc absorption. Both foods have been found to substantially decrease the absorption of zinc from high-zinc oysters.[23] The phytate in grains binds with zinc and inhibits its absorption, not only from the zinc in the grains themselves but also from zinc-rich foods that are eaten with them.

Although the effects of phytate on mineral absorption have been known for decades, many health professionals seem strangely unaware or unconcerned about them. Harold H. Sandstead, M.D., a zinc expert and prevention medicine and community health professor at the University of Texas, Galveston, summarized this situation well in a 1992 editorial.

> The evidence seems overwhelming that high intakes of fiber sources that are also rich in phytate can have adverse effects on mineral nutriture of humans. . . . In view of the [reviewed] data, it appears that some health promoters who suggest that U.S. adults should consume 30–35 g dietary fiber daily either have not done their homework or have simply ignored carefully done research on this topic.[24]

Other Antinutrients in Whole Grains

Quite a few other antinutrients are in whole grains, including alkylresorcinols, alpha-amylase inhibitors, and protease inhibitors. Most of these are believed to have evolved in grains as a defense mechanism—a way that grains could protect themselves from being eaten by insects and possibly animals and people. According to Cordain, these substances may be toxic, antinutritional, or somewhere in between. Little research has been done on these substances in humans. Cordain has summarized what is known about these substances in his paper:[25]

- In cell studies, alkylresorcinols (found in the highest amounts in rye and wheat) have been shown to stimulate increased production of platelet thromboxane, which promotes inflammation.

- In animal studies, chronic administration of alpha-amylase inhibitors (found in wheat and other grains) have been shown to induce adverse effects on pancreas cells and pancreatic overactivity.

- Alpha-amylase inhibitors also are known to be the cause of baker's asthma, an occupational allergy with a high prevalence in the baking industry. In addition, they may be important allergy-producing substances in wheat sensitivity.

- Protease inhibitors (found in all grains and legumes) inhibit the activity of digestive enzymes that help break down protein. The effect in humans of chronic low-level exposure to these substances is unknown, but an animal study found that these substances helped to cause pancreatic stress.

The intricate details concerning these substances aren't that important, and all these substances may not be harmful. However, so many potentially problematic substances are in whole grains that it should be a cause for concern.

Lectins

Lectins are glycoproteins (proteins with carbohydrate attached to them) and are considered the major antinutrient of food. Identified in wheat, corn, rye, barley, oats, and rice, lectins are found in higher concentrations in whole grains than in refined grains, and cooking doesn't break them down.

Lectins were originally identified by their ability to agglutinate or clump with red blood cells, but they actually can bind and interact with every single cell in the body.[26] This characteristic of lectins means that they have a high potential to interfere with the body's normal hormonal balance, metabolism, and health if they breach the protective barrier of the gut wall and enter the bloodstream.[27] Animal studies and human research suggest that this does indeed happen.

You'll learn in Chapter 6 that our gut is more permeable than once thought, and many factors can make a gut leakier than normal. Dietary lectins, it turns out, are one of those factors. The best-studied lectin is wheat germ agglutinin or WGA. In rats, WGA at high concentrations damages cells in the intestinal lining, interferes with digestion and absorption in the small intestine, and causes an imbalance in gut bacteria.

WGA also is rapidly transported across the gut wall into systemic blood circulation. In the human research done in this area, antibodies to WGA have been routinely found in healthy people and in people with celiac disease, a severe sensitivity to gluten. Other human research shows that peanut lectin appears in the blood one to four hours after people eat peanuts,[28] so it's virtually certain that lectins from both grains and legumes easily pass through the gut wall and into circulation.

Once they pass into circulation, lectins may fool the immune system into reacting to proteins that it shouldn't react to. This process is called molecular mimicry, and it sets the stage for developing autoimmune disorders, which I will cover after I tell you Marge's story.

Marge's Story

In 1994, Marge, a forty-five-year-old school teacher, began eating more whole grains and beans after she read a magazine article that touted their benefits. Marge noticed some initial digestive bloating but thought that was normal.

As time went on, Marge began to have on-and-off digestive trouble and mistakenly assumed her bloating and digestive upset might be caused from the meat and eggs she was still eating, so she gradually cut animal protein from her diet. A few months later she ran into someone at a vitamin shop who suggested that she try a high whole-grain, macrobiotic diet. At first enthusiastic about the diet, Marge abandoned it after six months when she started to develop noticeably achy and stiff joints.

While still avoiding meat and eating a lot of whole grains, Marge became increasingly concerned that she wasn't getting enough calcium and protein, so she added soy- and dairy-based protein powders, yogurt, soy foods, and a lot of cheese to her diet. Her joint achiness and inflammation only worsened.

Next, Marge guessed that she might be low in vitamins and minerals, so she began taking a multiple once-a-day supplement. Although this initially helped ever so slightly, her joint stiffness and inflammation continued and became so severe that she could sometimes barely bend her fingers. She decided to visit her doctor who diagnosed her with rheumatoid arthritis and prescribed a nonsteroidal anti-inflammatory drug. The medication gave her initial relief from her pain, but she didn't like the idea of taking a drug for the rest of her life. She also got the distinct impression that she had become increasingly sensitive to foods, but she couldn't really pin down exactly which foods were causing the problems.

As luck would have it, a work associate suggested that she try removing gluten (found in wheat, rye, barley, and oats) from her diet and adding fish and omega-3-enriched eggs for the valuable anti-inflammatory omega-3 fats they contained. Initially hesitant to try this advice, Marge analyzed her diet-health situation and realized that most of her health problems began after she started to eat so many whole grains (especially whole wheat products). It seemed reasonable that gluten could be the problem, so she cut it out of her diet. As a result, her joint inflammation and achiness lessened dramatically, and she felt better overall. Encouraged, she gradually added some omega-3-rich foods to her diet and this helped improve her condition as well.

After about a year of following a gluten-free diet, Marge felt better. However, her joints still ached and she was unable to get off the medication that had been prescribed for her. One of my clients, a friend she hadn't seen in years, recommended that she call me up for an appointment. I asked her how serious she was about wanting to go on the most therapeutic diet for her condition. She said she was very serious, so I gave her the final piece of the puzzle—to cut out all grains, legumes, yeast, and dairy products. She did, and her condition cleared up fairly quickly. With the help of her doctor, she was able to wean herself off the nonsteroidal anti-inflammatory drug that she was told she would need for the rest of her life.

The Lectin Connection to Autoimmune Diseases

Grains are the only foods known to be causative agents for at least two autoimmune diseases: celiac disease and dermatitis herpetiformis. You'll learn a lot more about these conditions in the next chapter. It's important to understand, though, that grains are also implicated in the development of virtually all autoimmune disorders. Among scientists who study diseases of ancient populations, it's generally believed that autoimmune diseases did not plague humans before they began including grains in their

A Simple Model of How
Autoimmune Diseases May Develop

Step 1: Lectins increase gut permeability and cause bacterial overgrowth, which allow undegraded protein fragments from food, bacteria, and viruses to pass through the gut wall, enter the bloodstream, and travel to various parts of the body.

Step 2: Once the protein fragments from food, bacteria, and viruses pass through a leaky gut and into circulation, they may fool the immune system because they share common characteristics with some body proteins.

Step 3: The immune system may not be able to distinguish self from nonself. It mistakes its own tissues for the protein fragments the tissues resemble and attacks them.

diets. Autoimmune diseases include rheumatoid arthritis (which leaves tell-tale signs in the fossil record), autoimmune thyroid disease, autoimmune liver disease, Crohn's disease of the bowel, ulcerative colitis, Type 1 diabetes, systemic lupus erythematosus, multiple sclerosis, psoriasis, Sjogren's syndrome (a dry-eye, dry-skin condition), and others, possibly including allergies, skin rashes, and asthma.

Lectins from not only grains but also legumes are believed to play several key roles in the development of autoimmune diseases. To illustrate the most likely scenario of how lectins are involved, let's take the example of rheumatoid arthritis.[29] Lectins begin the process by inducing structural changes in the intestine that increase gut permeability. They also help to cause bacterial overgrowth. These two factors allow passage of both undegraded proteins from food and proteins (antigens) derived from bacteria and viruses into circulation.

It turns out that protein fragments from grains, legumes, dairy foods, and yeast that pass into circulation have amino acid sequences that are the same or very similar to amino acid sequences in a variety of human tissues. When these protein fragments (whether from food or from viruses or bacteria) travel to tissues, the body mounts an attack on them but also ends up attacking its own tissues. That's because protein fragments in them look so much like the invaders, at least in people with certain genes. This same general concept appears to apply to all autoimmune diseases. Lectins act like a Trojan horse that allows invaders into the body.

To stop or at least reduce the autoimmune process in genetically susceptible people, eliminating foods that have proteins that look like those found in tissues—in other words, removing grains, legumes, dairy foods, and yeast from the diet—is the best nutritional strategy, along with using supplements to help heal the gut (which will be covered in Chapter 16). Many practitioners, including myself, have seen positive results with this type of diet therapy.

Some researchers might say the research is too preliminary to advocate a diet free of grains, legumes, dairy foods, and yeast for those with autoimmune diseases. I readily acknowledge that there is a great need for more research into the lectin connection to autoimmune diseases, and it is my hope that public interest in the problems with grains will spur accelerated scientific research. However, even with that, it will take scientists, optimistically, decades to iron out all the intricate details of how lectins are involved in different autoimmune diseases.

In the meantime, many people are suffering with autoimmune disorders. Standard medical care offers little to help those people, except for giving drugs such as nonsteroidal anti-inflammatory drugs (NSAIDs), which undoubtedly make the conditions worse because they are known to increase gut permeability. The most proactive thing a person with an autoimmune disease can do is extrapolate from the research and follow a dietary plan that has the best chance of reversing the autoimmune process. From a historical viewpoint, it makes sense that grains, dairy products, legumes, and yeast, which are the newest foods in the human diet, are the ones most likely to cause serious health problems. We simply haven't had adequate time to adapt to them, and the development of autoimmune diseases is living proof of that biological reality.

Researchers are correct in that very few clinical trials involving the elimination of some nongluten grains or beans have been conducted. However, research into the elimination of gluten grains (wheat, rye, barley, and possibly oats) has been quite extensive and the evidence is overwhelming that eliminating gluten grains is an absolute must for those with autoimmune diseases. Although not a true glycoprotein, gluten has lectin activity and causes plenty of health problems. In the next chapter, you'll learn about the gluten connection to everything from autism to infertility to some types of cancer.

CHAPTER 5

The Trouble with Gluten Grains

Of all the grains, wheat is the most problematic, and this is largely because it contains the most gluten. Gluten is a gluey collection of proteins also found in wheat cousins (spelt and kamut), rye, triticale (a wheat-rye hybrid), barley, oats, and an endless variety of processed foods. Bakers and food manufacturers love gluten—and praise the types of wheat that contain the most gluten—because it's the stuff that makes bread rise and puff up beautifully. However, what many consumers don't know is it's also the stuff that causes the health of many people to plummet, often in extremely insidious ways.

First, some basics. There are an amazingly wide variety of reactions that occur to gluten, but conventionally trained physicians only recognize celiac disease, the most serious type. (Celiac, pronounced seel-ee-ac, means abdominal.) Celiac disease is an autoimmune-type reaction in which the body reacts so strongly to gluten that it whittles away and flattens out the delicate lining of the small intestine, causing chronic malabsorption of nutrients. It historically has been characterized by diarrhea, bloating, acute abdominal pain, fatty stools, and often weight loss. In severe cases, celiac disease is life threatening, especially when it goes undiagnosed for years in children. This is still too often the case because physicians have been taught that celiac disease is very rare, believed to occur in only one in every 1,000 to 7,000 people.

Danielle's Story

In 1998, pro-football quarterback Rich Gannon and his wife Shelley became very worried. Their precious one-year-old daughter Danielle had been a fussy baby since birth, but she suddenly began crying all the time, developed extreme diarrhea, and began to lose weight. Her eyes, which had been bright and perky, became dull and sunken.

The Gannons knew something was very wrong and were alarmed, so they took Danielle in for test after test. Danielle was getting sicker and sicker, but she had to endure continually being poked, prodded, and scanned, and Rich and Shelley felt helpless to stop her suffering and were afraid she might die.

After months of no answers, a new doctor followed a hunch and did a few more tests. A blood screen and an intestinal biopsy confirmed that Danielle had celiac disease. Wheat and other common grains were making her sick, and the cure was simple: it didn't involve drugs or surgery or some type of organ transplant, only a change in diet.

Rich and Shelley were elated—that is, until they found out how difficult it was to avoid every little speck of wheat that's hidden in the average diet. Taking control of Danielle's diet and making sure it was entirely gluten free was a frustrating learning experience at first—Danielle would occasionally suffer relapses of poor health when she unexpectedly ate gluten in foods that her parents never suspected. But with so much at stake, the Gannons kept with it and eventually mastered the new routine. Today Danielle is a healthy, perky five-year-old, totally free of any signs of her illness as long as she doesn't inadvertently eat gluten.

The Changing Picture of Celiac Disease

Increased research and newly developed blood screening tests have led to shocking revelations. (Unfortunately, most physicians are too busy to stay up to date on the latest research.) First, celiac disease is very common: it's found in 1 in every 167 healthy children in the United States and 1 in every 111 healthy adults.[1] That makes it by far the single most common gastrointestinal disease, yet studies have found it even more common in other areas of the world. For example, the prevalence is 1 in 85 of the Finnish and 1 in 70 of the Italians in Northern Sardinia.[2]

Second, many people who have the disease don't have classic gastrointestinal celiac disease symptoms, and some don't have any symptoms at all. These people have *silent celiac disease*—a condition in which all the damage to the small intestine normally found in classic celiac disease is present without any obvious symptoms. As a result, some people go for years, often decades, without being diagnosed, while celiac disease slowly but silently chips away at their health, according to Alessio Fasano, M.D., director of the Center for Celiac Research at the University of Maryland. Their first indication of trouble may be finding out they have anemia, osteoporosis, or some type of autoimmune disease. Even worse, some people who develop these conditions have had celiac disease all along but have never been diagnosed with it: They never knew that gluten was the

---

The Prevalence of Celiac Disease in the United States[3]

Celiac disease is an immune system reaction to gluten that causes damage to the small intestine and malabsorption of nutrients, sometimes without any obvious symptoms but with severe complications. Recent research in the United States shows that celiac disease is a lot more common than ever imagined. It occurs in:

1 in every 167 healthy children

1 in every 111 healthy adults

1 in every 40 symptomatic children

1 in every 30 symptomatic adults

1 in every 12 first- and second-degree relatives of celiacs

real culprit behind their chronic health problems and that their health complaints likely could have been prevented had they known to eliminate gluten from their diets.

Victoria's Story

In 1978, at age twenty-six, Victoria, a graphic artist, went in to her doctor for her annual physical, and her blood work revealed a slightly low iron count. Her doctor prescribed an iron supplement and sent her on her way. A year later, Victoria came in for another physical. This time her blood iron count was a little lower. The doctor ran a few more tests and found nothing else unusual, so he thought there was nothing to be concerned about.

This pattern continued and worsened. Year after year, Victoria found that her blood iron count dropped lower and lower, and she became more and more exhausted. At one point, she was taking nine iron supplements a day, and yet on her next blood test, her iron levels barely registered! Frightened and frustrated, Victoria spent more money seeing specialists. They ran every test in the book on her and admitted they had no idea why she wasn't absorbing iron. Their only suggestion was that she go on an iron transfusion program in which iron was dripped into her veins for four hours every month—not a very fun proposition.

This process continued—believe it or not—for twenty years, and Victoria gave up trying to find an answer. Two years ago, though, her health worsened further. She became extremely pale and short of breath, and her fingernails started to curl up. She could barely bear the thought of going in for any more tests, but she did, this time to a gastroenterologist. A blood test and an endoscopy finally gave her an answer—she had celiac disease (silent celiac disease, in her case), something that could be corrected with a simple change in diet. She was relieved. "Thank God, it isn't cancer!" she thought to herself.

After starting a gluten-free diet, Victoria, unlike many celiacs, didn't feel much different for several months. It took quite a while for her body to heal and build up its iron stores, and she wondered if the trials and tribulations she went through to make sure that her diet was gluten free were worth it. Today, however, she knows it was. A little more than a year after her diagnosis, her iron count is almost back to normal, the color is back in her face, and she has more energy than she has had in decades.

Celiac Disease–Associated Conditions and Complications

These facts about celiac disease by themselves are shocking, but they're only a small piece of the story. Luigi Greco, M.D., of the University of Naples in Naples, Italy, has combed the published research and compiled a list of the symptoms, complications, and disorders associated with celiac disease, which he presented at the 9th International Symposium on Celiac Disease in the fall of 2000. The list of conditions—more than two hundred!—is truly mind-boggling. Celiac disease can wreak havoc in virtually any system of the body, not just the gastrointestinal tract but also the blood, the liver, the skin, the reproductive system, the endocrine glandular system, the immune system, and the brain and neurological system. An entire book could be written on the symptoms and complications of celiac disease, but here are just some of the highlights.

Autoimmune Diseases

Autoimmune diseases—conditions where the body literally turns on itself, attacking its own organs or tissues—are overrepresented in celiac disease. Some of the more common autoimmune diseases associated with celiac disease are insulin-dependent (Type 1) diabetes, dermatitis herpetiformis (a disease that causes blistering and intense itching of the skin), psoriasis, autoimmune thyroid disease, autoimmune liver disease, and connective tissue disease.

Italian researchers have found that the prevalence of autoimmune disorders in celiac disease is related to the duration of exposure to gluten. In other words, the longer people with celiac disease go undiagnosed and continue to eat gluten, the greater their likelihood of developing an autoimmune disease. Some people even develop multiple autoimmune disorders, such as insulin-dependent diabetes together with autoimmune

Common Symptoms of Celiac Disease

Celiac disease can be present with minor, nonspecific symptoms or without any noticeable symptoms. When symptoms are present, though, the following are some of the more common indicators:

Abdominal pain

Bloating

Diarrhea and/or constipation

Fatigue

Depression

Frequent canker sores

Dental enamel defects (vertical or horizontal grooves in teeth)

Iron-deficiency anemia

Low blood cholesterol

Low blood levels of zinc, vitamin D, vitamin K, and
    other nutrients

Short stature

Presence of autoantibodies (antibodies to self) in the blood

thyroid disease or connective tissue disease. Celiacs who are diagnosed and treated early, however, do not have an increased risk for autoimmune diseases. Unfortunately, most celiacs aren't diagnosed early: 77.5 percent of the time, the diagnosis of an autoimmune disorder is made first.[4]

So, what would happen if a gluten-free diet was started early in life, especially in those who are at greater risk for celiac disease or autoimmune diseases? No large-scale clinical trials have been done. However, insulin-dependent diabetes is one of the autoimmune diseases most closely associated with celiac disease, and preliminary results from a small trial in human subjects in Italy suggest that a gluten-free diet can protect against its development. The Gluten-Free Diabetes Prevention Trial study involved six people who were relatives of celiacs and had tested positive for elevated levels of autoantibodies involved in insulin-dependent diabetes. They were advised to go on a gluten-free diet, and after one year, only one of the six subjects still tested positive for the antibodies. In other words, these six subjects were all headed for insulin-dependent diabetes, but a gluten-free diet reversed that disease process and prevented them from developing it.[5] Although more research is needed, autoimmune processes seem to be going on in many areas of the body in celiacs, so a gluten-free diet likely protects against the development of many types of autoimmune diseases, at least in people who have celiac disease and don't know it.

Osteoporosis and Other Bone Diseases

Virtually every middle-aged woman I counsel is concerned about osteoporosis and wants to do what she can to prevent the disease, but none of my clients know about the gluten connection to osteoporosis. Osteoporosis and other bone diseases, such as rickets in children and osteomalacia in adults (caused from a vitamin D deficiency), are well-known consequences of celiac disease. In one recent study of eighty-six people newly diagnosed with celiac disease, two-thirds of the patients were found to have low bone mineral density and 26 percent were classified as having osteoporosis, the condition in which bones are more likely to break.[6]

The reasons why bone loss occurs in celiac disease are complex and poorly understood. Malabsorption of some nutrients, especially vitamin D, appear to be involved in many cases, but malabsorption of calcium is not always evident. Inflammatory compounds (cytokines) and hormonal dysregulation may also be at work.

Whatever the mechanisms involved, low bone mineral density is one of the major complications of celiac disease that goes undiagnosed. There is good news, though: for celiacs who are diagnosed and treated with a gluten-free diet, there is a significant improvement in bone mineral density in all ages, young and old, and the improvement is better than what can be accomplished with drug treatment of osteoporosis.[7] In addition, a study with celiac children found that by simply removing gluten from their diets, there was an increase in bone density greater than that seen in healthy children.[8]

Most of the improvement on a gluten-free diet occurs in the first year, but it's vital for celiacs to stay on a gluten-free diet. Although there are individual differences, the authors of one long-term follow-up study conclude: "According to our results, bone disease in celiac patients is cured in most patients during five years on a gluten-free diet."[9]

Infertility and Pregnancies of Poor Outcome

Undiagnosed celiac disease is one of the least-recognized reasons why couples can't conceive when trying to have a baby and why pregnancies result in unwanted outcomes, such as stillbirths, miscarriages, and low-birth-weight babies. A host of reproductive problems associated with celiac disease in both men and women set the stage for the inability to get pregnant or to carry a pregnancy to term. In men, impotence, underactive sexual development, and abnormal sperm forms and motility can occur.[10] In women, a delay in the beginning of puberty, amenorrhea (absence of menstrual periods), early menopause, recurrent miscarriages, and a reduced pregnancy rate often result.[11] The real mechanism by which celiac disease produces these changes is unclear, but malnutrition, such as zinc, folic acid, and iron deficiencies, are likely involved, as well as hormonal dysfunction.

Once again, the answer to this problem is withdrawing gluten from the diet. Correcting nutrient deficiencies with the use of supplements is also important. This approach has been able to restore fertility in both men and women. For example, in one study in which 845 pregnant women were screened, 12 were found to have celiac disease and 7 of those had unfavorable outcomes of pregnancy. However, after the women had been on a gluten-free diet for a year, six healthy babies were born with no problems.[12]

Celiac disease should be considered in all cases of unexplained infertility or pregnancies with poor outcome. In addition, it probably should be routinely tested for in *all* pregnant women in order to prevent unwanted, emotionally devastating consequences. As the authors of the above study state: "Celiac disease is considerably more common than most of the diseases for which pregnant women are routinely screened."[13]

Cancer

The risk of developing T-cell lymphoma, a small intestine cancer, is 40- to 100-fold (4,000 to 10,000 percent) greater in celiacs than in the general population.[14] In addition, celiacs also have an increased risk of developing other types of small intestine cancer and some types of esophageal and pharyngeal cancer.[15] This isn't surprising because in celiac disease, high levels of cell-damaging free radicals build up, nutrient deficiencies develop, and the immune system against cancer cells becomes impaired. However, if celiac disease is diagnosed before cancer becomes clinically evident and a gluten-free diet is then strictly followed, the risk of intestinal lymphoma decreases back to near normal levels in five years.[16] A gluten-free diet, therefore, helps prevent cancer in those who have celiac disease and don't know it. This is the most compelling reason to be screened for the disease, especially if you have a condition in which celiac disease is overrepresented, such as any of the conditions listed in this section. (You'll learn more about this in Chapter 7.)

The Spectrum of Gluten Sensitivity

As if the information on celiac disease wasn't compelling enough, it literally is just the tip of the iceberg of the different types of reactions that can occur to gluten. *Gluten sensitivity* is an umbrella term that includes classic celiac disease with gastrointestinal symptoms as well as the more recently recognized silent celiac disease. However, there's a whole spectrum of gluten sensitivity beneath the tip of the iceberg that is causing plenty of health problems but is getting little interest from researchers. You'll learn in this section that gluten sensitivity is far more prevalent than anybody could have ever imagined, and that a gluten-free diet is the treatment for gluten sensitivity, just as it is for celiac disease.

To learn more about gluten sensitivity, you need to first understand a little more about gluten. Gluten is a collection of proteins that consists of groups of long amino-acid chains (or peptides) called gliadins (the alcohol-soluble fragments) and glutenins (the water-soluble fragments). Researchers have focused on gliadin, especially one type of gliadin, as the culprit that starts the chain of events that lead to celiac disease. However, some research also suggests that a type of glutenin may be involved.

In any case, elevated levels of antibodies to gliadin have been used for decades as a way to help detect celiac disease. If the test comes back positive, then an intestinal biopsy is performed to confirm small intestine atrophy, which is necessary in order to receive a diagnosis of celiac disease from a doctor. (Today, additional, more celiac-specific blood tests are also used to help with the diagnosis.) However, there has always been a significant portion of the population—10 to 25 percent of North Americans, for example[17]—that has tested positive on the antigliadin blood antibody test but didn't have the damage to the small intestine that characterizes celiac disease. These people were told they didn't have celiac disease and were advised to continue to eat gluten.

Latent Celiac Disease

Unfortunately, researchers have now realized that some of the people who were told they didn't have celiac disease go on to develop celiac disease later on in life. At the time they tested positive for antigliadin antibodies, they had *latent celiac disease,* which then became active celiac disease years later because they continued to eat gluten. The exact percentage of gliadin-sensitive people who eventually develop celiac disease isn't known, but someone who is gliadin sensitive always runs the risk of developing celiac disease, with its more serious health consequences, later on.

In addition, many of those who test positive for gliadin sensitivity never develop celiac disease, but that doesn't mean they don't suffer from health problems. To the contrary, gluten sensitivity can wreak havoc on health in a wide variety of ways.

Malabsorption in Gluten Sensitivity

As one example, consider the research of Kenneth Fine, M.D., director and founder of the Intestinal Health Institute in Dallas, Texas, an internationally renowned gastrointestinal researcher and a pioneer in our understanding of gluten sensitivity. In an innovative study, Fine and his colleagues asked adults in a shopping mall—adults who didn't have gastrointestinal disease—if they would agree to have their blood drawn to be screened for a "a common nutritional syndrome." To avoid selection bias, the shoppers were not told the study was about gluten sensitivity. Ten percent (or 22) of the 221 volunteers who were tested showed high levels of antigliadin antibodies in their blood. Twenty of these 22 agreed to further testing and one woman tested positive for celiac disease. The other 19 did not. However, by using three different tests, Fine found that even without intestinal damage detectable on a biopsy, 50 percent of those who tested positive for gluten sensitivity had nutrient malabsorption and other abnormal tests of intestinal function that can cause illness.[18] This research shows that the function of the small intestine is affected well before its structure is.

New Research Indicates Prevalence of Gluten Sensitivity

Fine has developed a much more sensitive test that can detect cases of gluten sensitivity that aren't picked up with standard blood screens. (You'll learn more about this test in Chapter 7.) He also has been gaining more data about the genes that seem to be involved in gluten sensitivity. Here are the shocking results of his research so far:[19]

- The genes that seem to make a person susceptible to developing gluten sensitivity are exceedingly common: they're present in 60 to 70 percent of the population.

- At least 50 percent of the population is gluten sensitive.

Ten to 25 percent of the American population would be 28 to 70 million people. Fifty percent of the population would be 140 million. Whichever percentage you use, that's an unbelievable number of people whose immune systems are reacting to gluten and don't know it! Many of these people are likely not absorbing nutrients well and have increased intestinal permeability, which leads first to suboptimal health, then eventually to illness. In addition, the immune system is in overdrive, and that's likely affecting many other systems throughout the body.

The Iceberg of Gluten Sensitivity

Just as the tip of an iceberg is the only part visible above the water line, clinical celiac disease and silent celiac disease are the only types of gluten sensitivity diagnosed and recognized by conventional physicians. Hidden from view is a wide range of more subtle reactions to gluten that cause health disturbances and complications.

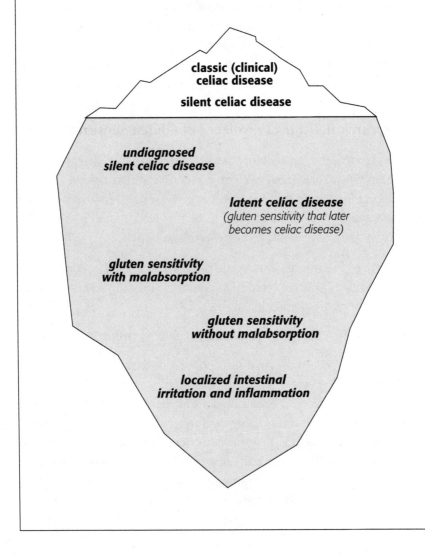

classic (clinical) celiac disease

silent celiac disease

undiagnosed silent celiac disease

latent celiac disease
(gluten sensitivity that later becomes celiac disease)

gluten sensitivity with malabsorption

gluten sensitivity without malabsorption

localized intestinal irritation and inflammation

Fatigue, depression, joint aches, bone pain, and abdominal and bowel complaints, such as gas, bloating, cramping, pain, irritable bowel, and diarrhea, appear to be some of the most common, everyday symptoms experienced by those with gluten sensitivity. Some people don't report any symptoms, but they almost always report improvements in their emotional and physical health that they hadn't expected after they follow a gluten-free diet for a few weeks or months.

Mary's Story

Mary began having minor health problems in her teens: bloating after meals, frequent canker sores, and blue moods, but she thought nothing of it. Out on her own when she went to college, she ate more junk food, especially a lot of pizza, and drank alcohol with her friends. Her abdominal bloating worsened, and she gained weight.

After she received her bachelor's degree, she started a job as a research assistant and began to feel depressed more often than not, which was perplexing because she was doing work she loved. She also developed a new symptom: occasional, debilitating migraine headaches, which would come on for no apparent reason.

Mary's bloating, canker sores, depression, and migraines continued on and off for five years, but none of these symptoms were extreme, so she just learned to live with them. However, after she turned thirty, she began to develop extremely itchy blisters on her legs. She saw several dermatologists who couldn't determine why these blisters developed, yet the blisters continued popping out occasionally and driving her crazy.

Finally, in 1995, at age thirty-two, Mary read a health book that mentioned that sensitivity to gluten can cause many unexplained health problems, so she tried cutting gluten out of her diet as an experiment. Within a week, her lifelong bloating and canker sores were gone, and she couldn't believe how much more energetic and brighter in spirit she was. She felt like it was a miracle that all her health complaints could be attributed to one common component.

However, like many people who find out they're gluten sensitive (especially when they don't have a firm diagnosis of celiac disease), Mary cheated a few times with some small amount of a wheat-based food. Each time she paid a price for it: bloating and depressed feelings came back with back with a vengeance. Though at times Mary wishes it weren't true, her body has made it very clear to her that avoiding gluten is what she must do.

Conditions Associated with Gluten Sensitivity

While gluten sensitivity can present itself in minor ways, particularly in the beginning of the disease process, it also can present itself through serious health problems, just like celiac disease. Remember: celiac disease is a part of gluten sensitivity, so any of the complications associated with celiac disease, such as autoimmune diseases, osteoporosis, infertility, and growth problems in children, can also occur in gluten sensitivity. (It appears that some people have certain genes or are exposed to certain environmental factors that cause gluten sensitivity to express itself as celiac disease and others don't.) However, there are plenty of disease conditions associated with gluten sensitivity that aren't found in celiac disease as often. Here are some of the more well-researched ones.

Colitis and Other Gastrointestinal Complaints

Colitis—inflammation of the colon, usually resulting in chronic diarrhea and cramping—can develop from a variety of factors, including gluten sensitivity. One type in particular, microscopic colitis (often diagnosed as collagenous colitis), is strongly linked to gluten sensitivity. Fine, who has studied microscopic colitis extensively, says that the damage done in the small intestine in celiac disease looks almost identical in a biopsy to the damage done in the large intestine in microscopic colitis. However, unlike celiac disease, Fine believes microscopic colitis is a secondary gluten-sensitive condition. In other words, it may develop from something else, such as an imbalance in good and bad bacteria in the colon, but once microscopic colitis develops, the immune system begins reacting to gluten, which makes the situation far worse. A gluten-free diet, along with use of supplements of good bacteria to correct the imbalance, is the only way to clear up the problem, according to Fine. Sometimes the standard treatment for microscopic colitis (bismuth subsalicylate, which is found in Pepto-Bismol) is also required.

A gluten-free diet has been reported to be helpful in a wide range of gastrointestinal difficulties, including conditions such as irritable bowel syndrome and stomach ulcers. Therefore, a gluten-free diet is worth a try in any case of gastrointestinal illness that hasn't been helped by other means. One recent study even found it beneficial in lessening diarrhea in patients with acquired immune deficiency syndrome (AIDS).[20]

Dermatitis Herpetiformis

Dermatitis herpetiformis is a well-known, gluten-sensitive skin disease, characterized by red bumps and blisters and intense itching, burning, and stinging, and it has long been associated with celiac disease. However, 20 to 25 percent of those with dermatitis herpetiformis never develop intestinal lesions, so they don't meet the criteria necessary to be diagnosed as having celiac disease. Nevertheless, dermatitis herpetiformis is associated with a higher risk for autoimmune diseases and intestinal lymphoma, and it responds well to a gluten-free diet: the rash slowly clears. If a gluten-free diet is discontinued, the rash returns.

Psoriasis

Psoriasis—a skin disease recognized by silvery scaling bumps and raised patches that flake, usually on the scalp, elbows, knees, back, and rear end—sometimes occurs in gluten sensitivity. In one study, 16 percent of patients with psoriasis had elevated antibodies to gliadin. All of the gluten-sensitive patients who followed a gluten-free diet for three months showed a significant improvement in their psoriasis. When an ordinary diet was resumed for a few months, more than half of the patients had their skin condition deteriorate.[21]

Nervous System Disorders, Dementia, and Frequent Unexplained Headaches

People with neurological disease of unknown cause have a much higher frequency of gluten sensitivity than the general population. In one study, 57 percent of the patients with neurological disorders of unknown origin—

especially ataxia (unsteady gait and shaky movements) and neuropathy (weakness and numbness of the limbs)—had high levels of antigliadin antibodies compared to only 12 percent in the control group.[22]

Other neurological conditions linked to gluten sensitivity include epilepsy, brain atrophy, and memory impairment in various ages, including people in their twenties and thirties.[23] Celiac disease is often diagnosed years or decades after early-stage dementia, so this is a compelling reason to detect gluten sensitivity early, before it advances and causes brain damage and dementia that can't be easily corrected.

Frequent unexplained headaches may be one of the first symptoms of gluten sensitivity and neurological disorders. Marios Hadjivassiliou, M.D., of the Royal Hallmashire Hospital, Sheffield, England, studied six female and four male patients with gluten sensitivity and headaches, some of whom also had unsteadiness or ataxia. All the patients had abnormal magnetic resonance imaging (MRI) tests that showed white matter characteristic of cerebral inflammation. Introduction of a gluten-free diet in nine of the patients resulted in complete relief from the headaches in seven patients and partial relief in the other two.[24]

How gluten sensitivity does its damage in neurological and cerebral disorders is still not known: it could be from nutrient deficiencies that develop (such as folic acid, vitamin B_{12}, and vitamin B_6 deficiencies), immune reactions to the gluten, or some direct toxic effect of the gliadin. Whatever the mechanism, it appears that the longer a gluten-sensitive individual with these conditions continues to eat gluten, the worse his or her condition becomes. Gluten-free diets haven't been found to work as well when neurological conditions are advanced.[25,26,27] Gluten-free diets are most therapeutic in the early stages of gluten sensitivity, before a lot of damage has been done.

Autism and Schizophrenia

Autism, which starts to develop by age two, is a disorder in which a young child doesn't develop normal social relationships, behaves in compulsive and ritualistic ways, and often communicates in a peculiar manner. Schizophrenia is a mental disorder that involves loss of contact with reality, delusions, hallucinations, impaired thinking, and inability to function at work or socially. High levels of antibodies to gluten and casein, a protein in milk products, have consistently been found in individuals with both these conditions,[28,29] and compelling research shows that a gluten-free, casein-free diet may dramatically reduce the symptoms present in these conditions.

According to Karl-Ludwig Reichelt, M.D., a pediatric researcher at the University of Oslo, Norway, and specialist in these conditions, autistic children and schizophrenics do not make enough peptidases, enzymes that break down the peptides (amino acid chains) of gluten and casein. As a result, these partially digested peptides from gluten and casein enter the bloodstream through a compromised gut wall, migrate to the brain, and adversely affect behavior and cognition. In the next chapter, you'll learn more about these partially digested gluten and casein fragments, which have been demonstrated to have opium- or morphinelike activity in the central nervous system. For now, understand that other factors may be involved in the development of these conditions. In autism, for example, vaccinations and mercury toxicity have been implicated, perhaps compromising gut integrity to allow gluten and casein peptides to pass into the bloodstream and do their dirty work on the central nervous system.

How helpful is a gluten-free, casein-free diet? In one 1995 study by Reichelt, he placed fifteen autistic children on such a diet for four years. All of them experienced improved social behavior, cognitive skills, and communication abilities, except when some temporarily resumed eating gluten- and casein-containing foods.[30] J. Robert Cade, M.D., of the University of Florida, Gainesville, has done similar research. In one of his studies, he found that 81 percent of the autistic children he treated with a gluten-free, casein-free diet displayed improvements in behavior.[31]

A gluten-free, casein-free diet also has had therapeutic effects in some schizophrenics.[32] In a classic study by the late medical researcher F. C. Dohan, M.D., routinely treated schizophrenics, who on admission were randomly given a grain-free, milk-free diet while on a locked ward, were discharged from the hospital about twice as quickly as control patients assigned to a high-grain diet. The beneficial effect disappeared when wheat gluten was secretly added to the grain-free diet.[33]

Susie's Story

Five-year-old Susie was a classic autistic child. She lived in her own little world—withdrawn, uncommunicative, and indifferent to other children. She behaved oddly, rocking her body back and forth, flapping her arms, and smelling and touching her hair often. She also had a great deal of fear and anxiety. She was terrified of hair washing, using pedestrians' crossings, and walking up and down steps, and she was in a special education program.

A few years ago, at the suggestion of a new doctor, Susie's parents put her on a diet free of all gluten and casein. Things started to change slowly but surely. After she had been on the new diet a little more than three months, she became more curious and gained interest in other children. As time went on, her fear started to lessen, her unusual behavior became less frequent, and her communication—both verbal and nonverbal—improved by leaps and bounds.

Today, two years after starting the gluten-free, casein-free diet, Susie is in many ways a normal seven-year-old girl. She smiles and laughs, reacts normally when spoken to, and likes getting hugs. She has learned to skip rope, swim, and ride a bicycle and engages wholeheartedly in games and play. She also participates in a club on a weekly basis and has a best friend she enjoys spending afternoons with.

Her improvement in school has been equally dramatic. After seven months on the diet, she moved from a special education class to an ordinary class. She has learned to read well. She also participates in class, asks questions, and eagerly talks with people she is close to about things she has seen or experienced. Both her teachers and her parents have noticed that her creativity, especially in painting and drawing, has skyrocketed.

Unanswered Questions About Gluten Sensitivity

Given the vastly different ways gluten sensitivity can express itself and the dramatic statistics regarding its prevalence, gluten sensitivity is an epidemic in hiding. It appears that millions of people are walking around with it and don't know it, even though they have health problems rang-

Does a Lack of Zinc Contribute to Some Cases of Gluten Sensitivity?

Zinc deficiencies or imbalances may play a role in some cases of gluten sensitivity. In my experience working with people who are gluten sensitive, I have found many to be low in zinc or overloaded with copper, mercury, or other heavy metals that depress zinc levels in the body. Zinc is needed to make metallothioneins that detoxify hazardous substances in the gastrointestinal tract and to make many peptidase enzymes that break down some proteins in grains. Low levels of zinc or high amounts of copper or mercury, therefore, may lead to lower amounts of these zinc-dependent enzymes and carriers, which may, in turn, promote or aggravate the development of gluten sensitivity.

ing from minor to serious that can be helped and often totally eradicated by making a simple change in their diet.

We've really just scratched the surface in our understanding of gluten sensitivity and how the condition does all the damage it does. As one last bit of food for thought, consider that a small study in *The Lancet* reported that high-wheat-gluten diets can alter the normal lining of the small intestine and cause intestinal lesions in healthy people.[34] This is likely because of lectins,[35] which, you learned in the last chapter, alter gut permeability, but the implications are startling. It might mean that very few people—or perhaps none of us—are safe from the detrimental effects of gluten if we eat enough of it and are exposed to other undetermined environmental factors—perhaps stress, viruses, or certain drugs—which may increase our susceptibility.

The amount of gluten used in that small study showed that the adverse effect on healthy individuals' intestinal linings was 40 grams per day. The average American eats 18 grams of gluten per day.[36] Some Americans eat less, but many people—especially those on low-fat, high-carbohydrate diets, grain-based vegetarian diets, or typical teenage junk-food diets—eat considerably more. If you think of the typical teenager who chows down on pizza, pasta, and sandwiches and snacks on pretzels, muffins, bagels, breakfast bars, cookies, and crackers, he or she could probably very easily reach the 40 grams per day mark. In addition, it's unlikely that 40 grams is a magical cutoff point. We probably all have different tolerances for gluten, and some of us probably develop problems with much less.

Remember, also, that our distant ancestors ate essentially no gluten, and even after the dawn of agriculture, the majority of mankind didn't live on gluten-containing grains. While some of us probably tolerate gluten better than others, it may be that none of us are genetically programmed to thrive on large amounts over a long lifetime.

Until more research is done and more questions are answered, all of us need to become more aware of the dangers of gluten and evaluate whether this common component of the North American diet is the culprit behind our health problems. This book will guide you in that discovery. In Chapter 7, you'll learn how to evaluate your sensitivity to gluten. Later in the book, you'll learn how you can enjoy tasty foods without gluten, if you need to eliminate it from your diet. In the next chapter, you'll learn more about different immune reactions that can occur to grains and how grain allergies can lead to strong cravings and even addictions.

CHAPTER 6

Grain Allergies and Cravings and Genetically Engineered Foods

When most people think of food allergies, they think of immediate, obvious reactions such as breaking out in hives thirty minutes after eating strawberries or the throat closing up shortly after eating peanuts. It's true that in traditional allergy circles, these strong, quick reactions are considered the only true allergies to food—and they can sometimes occur from eating grains such as wheat—but they're rare. The vast majority of adverse reactions that occur to food (and grains in particular) are more delayed in nature and are therefore much harder to pin down.

Just as most types of gluten sensitivity go unrecognized by traditionally trained physicians, so, too, do delayed food allergies, which I will also refer to as food sensitivities. These types of reactions (in which IgG antibodies instead of IgE antibodies are involved) cause a wide range of adverse symptoms, just as gluten sensitivity does. Perhaps more baffling, a third to half of all people who have these reactions actually end up craving the very food that is causing them health problems. Wheat in particular is a common food allergen, addictant, and trigger to cravings, and there are real physiological reasons why this occurs, which you'll learn about shortly.

Characteristics of Delayed Food Allergies

Delayed allergies can develop to any food, but they almost always involve commonly eaten foods. In the United States, wheat, dairy, and corn products are eaten in hidden forms at almost every meal, so these are the most likely culprits. Food sensitivities produce slow responses to food: symptoms can show up a few hours to a few days after the food is eaten. Because of the time lag, people usually don't make the connection between the food and the symptoms.

Food sensitivities also begin insidiously and progress slowly. They might start with an allergy to one food, such as wheat, which causes a headache hours later. Because a headache can be caused by so many things, many people shrug it off and never attribute it to the wheat they ate. Time passes and other symptoms pop up, but they usually don't make the connections between the symptoms and the wheat, so they keep eating it. The body adapts to repeated assaults from the problem food, but it grows tired from dealing with the constant stressor. Symptoms, in turn, often get stronger. Eventually new sensitivities, with new symptoms, develop. When people eliminate the problem food or foods for a week or longer, many of the symptoms they had been experiencing on a routine basis go away, and if they reintroduce the foods, the body's reactions to them are usually much more dramatic and noticeable.

Ryan's Story

As an infant, Ryan developed colic and recurrent middle-ear infections. During the next five years of his life, asthma became a problem for him. An astute allergist traced this ailment to an allergy to wheat and cow's milk, and when his mother made sure to keep these foods out of Ryan's diet, his asthma cleared up.

When Ryan entered first grade, he began drinking milk and eating wheat products every day at school. Strangely enough, it seemed as if he had outgrown his allergy or had adapted to the regular intake of these foods because they no longer caused him noticeable symptoms. He loved and craved milk and wheat because they made him feel good.

Common Symptoms of Delayed or Hidden Food Allergies[1]

Delayed food allergies or food sensitivities, which often occur from eating wheat, corn, and other common foods, can cause a wide range of symptoms, depending on the individual. The most common indicators are:

- **Tiredness or even exhaustion**, particularly after meals, after a full night's sleep, or combined with other food sensitivity symptoms, such as depression or gastrointestinal upset

- **A tendency to gain or lose more than a couple of pounds a day**

- **Puffiness, swelling, or dark bags under the eyes**

- **Digestive ailments**, including bloating, flatulence, constipation and/or diarrhea, upset stomach, or abdominal pains or cramps

- **Excess mucus formation** characterized by a chronically congested nose, postnasal drip, a runny nose, frequent infections, sneezing fits, or excessive phlegm

- **Chronic pain** in the form of rheumatoid arthritis, muscle aches and pains, or sore, stiff joints

- **Headaches**, especially cluster and migraine headaches

- **Emotional, mental, and behavioral symptoms**, such as mood swings, unexplained irritability, panic attacks, hyperactivity, inability to concentrate, and depression for no apparent reason

Pizza, pasta, and Mexican food were his favorites, and he ate these foods all through his grade school, teenage, and college years.

Toward the end of college, Ryan developed a series of unexplained ailments—abdominal cramps and diarrhea and unexplained depression that would come and go. He saw numerous doctors over the next few years, all to no avail. Then a coworker mentioned in passing information about a delayed food allergy test she had done, and he decided to have the test done, too. The test revealed sensitivities not only to wheat and dairy, but also to tomatoes and beef. These were two foods he almost always ate in combination with wheat and dairy (such as cheeseburgers with ketchup, Philly cheesesteak sandwiches, and pasta with meatballs, tomato sauce, and cheese).

Avoiding all four foods was a real struggle for the first five days. Ryan had built all his habits around these foods, and he felt physically and emotionally uncomfortable eliminating them. However, a week into his revised diet, his abdominal troubles cleared, the depression lifted, and he felt like a new man.

The Changing Picture of Food Allergies

Delayed food allergies aren't taken seriously by many conventional physicians for many reasons. For one thing, no drug can cure or alleviate the symptoms of food allergies. The only solution is dietary, and unfortunately, most physicians aren't well schooled in nutrition.

Also, cause-and-effect thinking tends to rule medicine: this causes that. Each disease is supposed to have a specific set of symptoms and a specific cause. According to Dr. Jonathan Brostoff, a physician and professor of allergy and environmental health from University College London Medical School, and writer Linda Gamlin in their book *Food Allergies and Food Intolerance*, this line of thinking began in the 1860s and 1870s with the germ theory of disease and has dominated medical education ever since. Food sensitivities fly in the face of this type of thinking. The symptoms attributed to delayed food allergies cover an astoundingly wide range, from minor to severe and can affect every system in the body. There is no defining symptom common to all. A sensitivity to a food such as wheat can cause joint aches in one person; gas, bloating, and abdominal cramping in another; depression and nasal congestion in a third; and all of the above in a fourth. Also, the same symptoms can be brought on by different foods in different people.

How can illness from food allergies be so nebulous? It's because multiple factors contribute to the development of food allergies. Many different systems are involved in protecting us from food allergies, and it's likely that more than one malfunction in the body has to happen for them to develop. Since each person has a unique combination of circumstances leading up to his or her illness, this would explain why the symptoms and severity of illness in delayed food allergies run such a gamut.

New Insights into Digestion and Immunity

The digestive system is, obviously, the main system that deals with food. The traditional view is that enzymes in the mouth, stomach, and small intestine break down food into small molecules—sugars from complex carbohydrates and amino acids from protein. These molecules are absorbed into the bloodstream, but immune cells don't react to them because they're too small. Larger molecules that could cause trouble supposedly never get through an impregnable gut wall.

Research in the last several years and decades has debunked this view in several ways. First, chains of amino acids called peptides are absorbed by the small intestine more often than single amino acids. Undigested or partially digested food molecules regularly get into the bloodstream after a meal not only in food-allergic people but also in healthy individuals.[2,3,4] In fact, specialized areas of the gut wall actually sample intact food molecules from the gut contents to determine how the body should respond to them.

Common Malfunctions in Digestion

All of us have a gut that's a little more permeable than has long been believed. However, people who have food allergies have greater intestinal permeability, or a leakier gut, than nonallergic people.

So, what causes the intestinal lining to break down? A lot of common factors in our modern-day world. As you learned in Chapter 4, lectins from whole grains and beans are one overlooked factor. Other major contributors are drinking a lot of alcohol, overusing antibiotics and nonsteroidal anti-inflammatory drugs (NSAIDs), such as aspirin, ibuprofen, and prescription NSAIDs, and eating gluten and other foods a person is sensitive to. In some people, a milk allergy can cause the same type of overt damage to the small intestine that celiac disease does.[5]

Sometimes a person develops a viral, bacterial, parasitic, or yeast infection and is never quite the same afterward. The immune system attacks the invader and produces inflammation, which in turn makes the gut wall leakier. Other contributing factors include premature birth, early exposure to whole foods in infants, deficiency of beneficial intestinal bacteria (often due to overuse of antibiotics), and low levels of glutamine, the primary fuel for the intestinal lining, which is depleted during extreme stress and traumas. Types of extreme stress that can cause a depletion include viral infections, long periods of fasting, injuries, surgery, high fever, and exhausting endurance sports.

Given that virtually everyone runs into at least one of these factors sometime in life, it's probably common to have periods of increased intestinal permeability, with greater amounts of large, partially digested food molecules seeping into the bloodstream. Even so, the body has an extraintestinal, second level of digestion in the liver that serves as a backup detoxifier against the toughest foods for the body to break down—disulfide-bond-rich foods, such as gluten and milk protein. Once food fragments go through the intestinal lining, into the bloodstream, and then into the liver, high concentrations of a protein-cracking digestive enzyme in the liver (called thioredoxin) split the disulfide bonds in gluten and milk protein fragments and eliminate the allergic potential of these foods. According to James Braly, M.D., an expert in delayed food allergies and gluten sensitivity, healthy people probably have marginally leaky guts, with a trickling of large food fragments into the bloodstream, on a regular basis. However, their immune systems work well at engulfing and digesting the food fragments, and their livers work well at breaking down the most highly allergenic ones, so the food fragments don't cause reactions.

In allergic people, though, a number of things could be happening. People who are genetically predisposed to being allergic to disulfide-bond-rich foods, such as gluten and dairy, may have low levels of digestive enzymes in the liver, just as people who have lactose intolerance have low levels of lactase. Perhaps because of exposure to excessive amounts of chemicals, drugs, or alcohol, their liver detoxification system is taxed and may not be able to perform its additional digestive functions very well. Food-allergic people also almost always have leakier guts than normal, so that means there's a flood of polypeptides (large chains of amino acids) into the bloodstream. Perhaps the digestive enzymes and detoxification enzymes in the liver just can't keep up with all it needs to detoxify. There's also evidence that allergenic foods suppress release of gut hormones in a sensitive person, which in turn suppresses production of some digestive enzymes.[6,7,8] If people eat food allergens and this in turn suppresses digestive function, that also would cause the liver to have to work harder.

The bottom line: digestive enzyme deficiencies, a leaky gut wall, and an overworked liver detoxification system or immune system are all important factors in the development of food sensitivities. While some of us may be more genetically at risk for food allergies than others, modern-day contributing factors, such as the use of many common drugs or exposure to chemicals such as pesticides, leave us all susceptible to developing several chinks in the multisystem armor that protects against the development of food sensitivities.

The Many Components in Wheat That Can Cause Allergies

When a person has a sensitivity to wheat, he or she could be reacting to one or more of many different potential allergenic components in wheat, including:[9,10,11,12]

- Gliadins (of which there are forty different types)
- Glutenins (of which there are forty different types)
- Albumins
- Globulins

The Prevalence of Food Sensitivities

Just how common are delayed food allergies? Estimates have ranged from 10 to 60 percent of the population. The late Theron Randolph, M.D., one of the fathers of modern allergy research, called delayed food allergies "the most common undiagnosed illness in medicine."

Keep in mind that gluten sensitivity is a classic example of a food sensitivity, except instead of reacting to just one food, the body reacts to the collection of proteins called gluten, found in wheat, rye, and barley. One of the subfractions of gluten, alpha-gliadin, appears to be the primary component that causes sensitivities, but there are many other components in wheat a person can react to. Sensitivities also can occur to other grains and many other foods. Given that gluten sensitivity affects 10 to 50 percent or more of the population, it seems likely that food sensitivities affect a higher percentage of the population (almost always without people's knowledge).

Food Allergy-Addictions

One of the more perplexing aspects of food sensitivities is the phenomenon of food addiction. This is a condition in which people ironically feel a physical and emotional need for the very foods they're allergic to. In the course of some allergic reactions, the body produces narcotic-like substances, including feel-good endorphins, which elicit a temporary "high" and a short-lived amelioration of symptoms. Consciously or not, food-allergic individuals begin eating more and more of these foods, and then start including a daily dose of their problem foods to temporarily feel better and prevent uncomfortable symptoms of withdrawal. If they go too long without eating their favorite foods, they develop cravings and experience withdrawal. In time, food addicts find they need to eat large portions of their favorite food—for example, several plates of pasta—to get the same hit.

Although the concept may initially sound far-fetched, addictive eating as an aspect of food allergies has been observed repeatedly and reported in respected medical journals. Any practitioner who nutritionally counsels people on a regular basis, including myself, knows that it's a real phenomenon that can't (or at least shouldn't) be ignored.

The Price of Eating Food Allergens

There's a big price to pay for habitually eating allergy-producing foods and staying in a stimulated but relatively symptom-free state of health. According to Theron Randolph and Ralph W. Moss, Ph.D., authors of the classic book, *An Alternative Approach to Allergies*, the body's ability to adapt to these constant reactions eventually falters and breaks down. Foods or beverages that used to make the person feel good lose their punch, and the body can no longer hold withdrawal symptoms at bay. The body also can't easily correct or balance the disease condition that has been going on for years. A chronic state of illness involving multiple organs and tissues and sometimes incapacitating symptoms can then develop. It's far more difficult to treat food sensitivities in this state than in their earlier, less severe states.

Hooked on Gluten, Corn, and Dairy Products?

Research investigating the occurrence of druglike substances in common foods over the past few decades has shed new light on the mechanisms behind food allergy-addictions. Studies have revealed that cereal grains, especially wheat, maize, and barley, and dairy products contain opioid substances called exorphins.[13,14,15] Opioid substances have a very similar sequence of amino acids to those in our natural endorphins and apparently can bind to endorphin receptors in the brain. They also have a very similar sequence of amino acids to those in addictive, narcotic-like drugs—exorphins literally mean morphine-like molecules that come from the outside environment. In simple terms, exorphins produce narcotic-like and mood-altering effects and can be addictive.

What does all this mean? Many of us may be getting low doses of narcotic-like drugs from eating regular amounts of the wheat-, corn-, and dairy-based foods Americans have become obsessed with. In the beginning, people may get a false sense of comfort and well-being from eating these foods. (It's interesting that in their initial consultation with me, several new clients of mine have told me that pasta is a "comfort food" for them.) Also, as you'll recall from Chapter 2, some researchers have proposed this grain-induced reward of a sense of comfort as the real reason why humans gave up their hunting-and-gathering life for an agricultural existence.

If allergies to gluten, corn, and milk develop and worsen, these foods begin to have more adverse, druglike effects. Food-allergic individuals, you might remember, don't digest food very well, and they also tend to have greater intestinal permeability than normal. That means that narcotic-like exorphins (partially digested compounds in gluten grains, corn, and milk) flood the bloodstream. If exorphins get to receptors before they are broken down by enzymes (especially protein-cracking enzymes in the liver, the backup to the digestive system), their druglike effects intensify. When you add the narcotic-like effects of exorphins from gluten, corn, and milk to the narcotic-like effects of internally created opioids (endorphins) that are released during allergic reactions, you can get a double-strength opioid effect. The stage is set for addictive eating behavior.

New information continues to be discovered and researched, which adds missing pieces to the puzzle of food addiction. For example, people with the most severe type of gluten sensitivity have been found to have low levels of serotonin, dopamine, and norepinephrine, three key brain neurotransmitters.[16] A gluten-free diet raises these levels back to normal. Researchers have theorized that exorphins cause deficiencies of these hormones—and serotonin and dopamine are particularly important for maintaining steady moods, controlling the appetite, and preventing cravings. If many people with gluten sensitivity or with food sensitivities to grains and milk have similar changes in their brain neurochemistry, this could be another way in which exorphins from common foodstuffs contribute to strong food cravings and the tendency to overeat favorite foods.

Suzanne's Story

Suzanne's eating habits were out of control. The thirty-two-year-old advertising executive tried to be careful with her diet, but she literally was always hungry.

Suzanne had pasta for dinner virtually every night because it was quick and easy to make. Her food diary, like many others I've seen, included constant fixes of wheat—a bagel here, pretzels there, sandwiches for lunch, and low-fat cookies for a small treat almost every afternoon and evening. She admitted to me that these foods used to make her feel incredibly good, but they didn't have the same effect they used to. She always wanted more, and she had gained fifteen pounds in the last year.

Before coming to see me, Suzanne tried to cut down on the portions of her favorite foods, but that strategy made things worse. She developed such strong cravings for the foods she loved that she would end up bingeing on a variety of wheat-based sweets.

I looked over her food diary and saw wheat and sugar as clear problem foods for her. They were eaten in so many different forms at so many different times throughout each day that I counseled her to avoid them and eat more lean meat and vegetables. I warned her that she might initially feel very strong cravings but that she should hang in there with this new diet for one week as an experiment, then contact me after that to let me know how she was doing.

A week and a half later, Suzanne called me up. She said that during the first few days, she felt like a drug addict going through withdrawal. The fourth evening was particularly difficult for her. However, when she awakened the next morning, she felt totally different: calm and centered, well rested, not hungry, and interested in the activities she was going to do instead of food!

Since that time, Suzanne has tried eating wheat from time to time but has realized that she has a strong allergy-addiction to it that's tough to crack. She likes being in control of her food habits instead of having food control her. She also likes having her trim figure back. To Suzanne, avoiding wheat and sugar are small prices to pay for these benefits.

The Food Sensitivity Connection to Weight Problems

Besides provoking countless health complaints, food sensitivities also are an unsuspected contributor to overweight conditions. When hidden food allergens are identified and eliminated, weight reduction is a common consequence—and this usually occurs without caloric restriction. Food allergy specialist James Braly, M.D., at one time had two clinics known for their ability to help people lose weight the food allergy elimination way. He has literally seen thousands of people easily drop pounds by removing their hidden food allergens—usually by eating more food, not less—when nothing else seemed to work.

Other health professionals who treat delayed food allergies, including bariatric (weight loss) specialists who are in the know, have noticed this same phenomenon. Clinical experiments have also shown this effect. For example, in one study involving forty-four rheumatoid arthritis patients who underwent an elimination diet, the patients, on average, lost about ten pounds during the six-week trial.[17] (Three-quarters of the patients also said their joint pain and stiffness felt better or significantly better at the end of the diet, and many experienced striking improvements.) The patients in this study were taken off all grains, milk products, eggs, and other commonly eaten foods for a week. Then the excluded foods were reintroduced, one at a time, and any that caused a flare-up of symptoms (such as wheat) were not eaten again.

The Role of Inflammatory Substances

Hidden food allergies probably contribute to being overweight in several different ways. First, they can cause water retention and water weight gain. After partially digested food compounds pass through a compromised intestinal lining into the bloodstream and to tissues, they cause irritation and inflammation. The body tries to reduce the irritation by retaining water, which dilutes the concentration of the offending material. As long as people consistently eat food allergens, they often hold on to water weight. Looking puffy or feeling bloated are common signs that a person might have food sensitivities.

Inflammatory substances that are released during food allergic reactions also affect weight control. Some chemicals involved in food allergies may inhibit metabolism, and prostaglandin E2, which is also released, inhibits the body's ability to burn fat stores, according to Braly. Food allergies, therefore, may diminish the body's ability to burn fat, a process known as lipolysis.

The Role of Opioids

As already discussed, food allergies often lead to food addictions, which sabotage weight control. Because partially digested compounds in common food allergens act like morphinelike opioid drugs, eating food allergens creates a temporary "high" initially, but when that feeling wears off, we crave our allergens again to get another "fix" of that euphoric feeling. Eventually we eat our food allergens so often that we become physiologically and psychologically addicted to them. If we try to eat less of the foods we're addicted to (as we usually do when we restrict calories to lose weight), that's like asking an alcoholic to have one small glass of alcohol a day. We often develop such uncontrollable cravings for our favorite foods that we end up bingeing on them. Binge-eating, in turn, encourages weight gain.

Opioid peptides in excess also increase appetite and decrease metabolism.[18] This applies to opioid peptides normally produced by the body as well as those found in partially digested compounds in grains and milk. This means if we're allergic to gluten grains, corn, and milk, the more we eat them, the more likely it is we will overeat. Even if we use willpower to somehow ignore our increased appetite and actually eat fewer calories, we still might gain weight if we continue to consume food allergens. That's because the body's calorie-burning efficiency could be diminished, and when excess calories aren't burned off, they're stored as fat.

The Weight Control Benefits of Eliminating Food Allergens

Eliminating food allergens, therefore, can conceivably offer many benefits: it can clear up bloating and water retention, help overcome food cravings and addictions, and boost metabolism and fat-burning lipolysis, at least in some people. Eating a widely varied, nonallergenic diet seems to be an unsuspected key for getting excess weight off and keeping it off, especially in people who have tried numerous other approaches without success.

Kim's Story

Kim, a forty-two-year-old housewife, came to see me because she was, in her words, "a mess." She had fatigue, abdominal bloating, dark circles under her eyes, frequent postnasal drip, sinus problems, painful menstrual periods, strong premenstrual cravings and mood swings, on-and-off skin rashes, and joint and muscle pain. She didn't mention it as a problem, but she was also about forty pounds overweight.

Given that Kim had so many clear signs of allergies, I suggested she have a blood test for delayed food allergies, along with a gluten sensitivity test. The gluten sensitivity test came out positive and her food allergy test showed sensitivities to wheat, rye, barley, oats, corn, milk, potatoes, a number of beans, and yeast (found in bread, vinegar, alcohol, and other fermented foods). I counseled her on how to whip up tasty meals without these foods, and she embarked on her personalized elimination diet.

One by one, her symptoms lessened or disappeared. Her abdominal bloating—something she had just learned to live with—cleared up within a few days. Her sinus problems and postnasal drip gradually abated, and two months after beginning her diet, she noticed that her premenstrual symptoms and menstrual periods were much less difficult.

Surprisingly, she started to easily lose weight, a bonus she simply wasn't expecting. She told me that she had tried countless diets and exercise programs and had lost hope that she would ever get rid of the excess weight. She never expected to find a program that would get both her health and her weight back in order at the same time, and she thanked me profusely for putting her on the right track. Within about six months, she was back to the size she was in college, and she was relieved of most of the complaints she came to see me about.

The Health Dangers of Genetically Engineered Foods

No discussion of either allergies or the problems with grains would be complete without also talking about genetically engineered (GE) foods, also called genetically modified foods. Would you like some pesticide in your corn? How about a heavy dose of lectins in your potatoes? Care for some fish genes in your tomatoes? That's exactly what genetically engineered foods do.

Dubbed "Frankenstein foods" or "Frankenfoods" by Europeans, genetically engineered foods are created when scientists implant genes from bacteria, viruses, insects, fish, and other living things into other species to give new traits to the recipient. Any way you cut it, this splicing and dicing is a sophisticated-sounding way of scientists playing God. Just about every other time people have fooled with mother nature—from refining sugar to using DDT as a widespread pesticide—they have gotten themselves into big-time trouble. With bioengineering, the results are likely to be worse because scientists are manipulating the very fabric of life.

Europeans are up in arms over these heavily tinkered foods and have vehemently protested their introduction into the food supply. Americans, on the other hand, seem rather uninformed and naive about GE foods and often put them in grocery carts without knowing it. This section gives an overview on the subject, with specific focus on the many problems that have surrounded genetically engineered corn.

The New Wrinkle in the Allergy Story

Transferring genes from viruses, bacteria, and other organisms surely will lead to unintended health consequences, especially for those with allergies. The DNA in genes directs the production of proteins—each gene makes not one protein, but more than one—and proteins are the common sources of human allergies. In addition, the gene that's inserted may attach in the middle of another gene and interfere with the normal functioning of the cell. It could even damage the DNA of the host, creating foods that contain allergens or toxins that people have never consumed before.

Very little human safety data on GE foods has been conducted, but there's already evidence to show that splicing DNA from one organism into another can turn a nonallergenic food into an allergy-producing food. Several years ago, a biotech seed company tried to change the protein content of soybeans by adding a gene from the Brazil nut. Researchers at the University of Nebraska, Lincoln, found that people with a sensitivity to Brazil nuts (who didn't have a sensitivity to soybeans) became allergic to the genetically engineered soybean.[19] Fortunately, based on those findings, the company discontinued the development of the soybean, but "the next case could be less ideal, and the public less fortunate," according to a companion editorial in the same issue of *The New England Journal of Medicine*.[20]

The above study concerned IgE allergies—the immediate, obvious kinds that are not common. Genetically engineered foods with drastically altered proteins will also surely contribute to IgG-mediated, delayed food allergies. As mentioned, delayed food allergies affect far more people, are harder to track down, and probably develop for a variety of reasons, including a deficiency of digestive enzymes or an overtaxed detoxification or immune system.

Consider what would happen if an allergic person ate some corn—which is a common allergen to begin with—and the corn was altered to include its own pesticide using a bacterium carrier. The body would then have three toxic invaders to deal with. This triple allergy threat would undoubtedly make the original sensitivity to corn much worse. Over time, it would probably also be enough to overload the body's defense system in those who aren't allergic to corn, precipitating the development of a corn sensitivity or some other type of intolerance.

Let the Buyer Beware: The StarLink Corn Example

The example described above may have already happened. A type of genetically engineered corn known as StarLink was approved by the Environmental Protection Agency (EPA) in 1998 for use as animal feed but not for human consumption because tests showed properties indicating it might cause allergies. (Unfathomably, the EPA didn't seem concerned about our eating animals or products from animals that eat unapproved GE foods.) Aventis, the company that produced StarLink, was supposed to make sure farmers segregated this corn from non-GE corn, but it didn't. Consequently, StarLink found its way into the human food supply. Two brands of taco shells—a Safeway house brand and Taco Bell brand made by Kraft Foods, a Philip Morris company—were found to contain Star-

Link corn. Nationwide recalls of these products were then issued, but not before reports came in to environmental groups and the FDA from people who said they got sick or suffered allergic reactions after eating the taco shells.

Fortunately, the EPA revoked the license it had given Aventis, and StarLink corn can no longer be planted for any agricultural purpose at all. However, this example highlights the fact that the bioengineering industry has gotten the regulations it wanted from Washington—not very strict ones. The industry also is essentially policing itself—and not doing a very good job of it. If the StarLink situation can happen, a similar situation can easily happen with other genetically engineered foods not approved for human consumption. But GE foods in general don't sound safe, whether they're approved by the FDA or not.

Other Alarming Aspects of Genetically Engineered Foods

StarLink corn is one of several genetically modified corn strains known as BT corn, so named because they contain a gene from the *Bacillus thuringiensis* (BT) bacteria. It causes the corn to produce a toxin that kills insects. Although BT is a highly effective pesticide long used by organic growers, BT corn and other BT plants have a little pesticide in every cell— an unsettling thought if you're eating those plants. In addition, the industry's own scientists believe that it's just a matter of time—perhaps three to five years—before BT-resistant insects develop. Then organic growers will lose a powerful pest control, and conventional growers may increase their use of chemical pesticides.

Evidence already exists that GE foods are a threat to the environment and to wildlife. A now-famous laboratory study by Cornell University researchers found that monarch butterfly larvae died after eating milkweed dusted with genetically modified corn pollen containing the BT pesticide. Milkweed, the monarch's primary food source, commonly grows alongside corn. Other studies with genetically modified foods have found harmful effects on ladybugs, green lacewings, and honey bees, which are all beneficial insects. Researchers also fear that once GE species cross-pollinate with their wild counterparts and with weeds, the safety of organic crops will be threatened, and a species of pesticide-resistant superweeds might be created.

Protect Yourself from Genetically Modified Foods: Buy Organic

You may think genetically engineered foods are bad but, because you're not actively seeking them out, they don't affect you. Wrong. If you're buying foods in a regular supermarket (especially corn products, soy foods, potatoes, and tomatoes), you're probably already unknowingly purchasing and eating GE foods.

In a situation that smells fishy to anyone with common sense, the FDA has chosen not to classify alien genes as food additives and therefore does not require that GE foods be labeled. Consequently, more than half the foods in regular grocery stores today are believed to contain some genetically modified ingredients, but consumers have no way of knowing which foods contain them.

The only surefire defense at this point is to buy certified organic products. Buying organic is something I highly recommend to safeguard your health (especially against the development of allergies), not to mention to help protect our environment. There are also a few companies, generally companies that make corn-based products found in health food stores, that specify that their products do not contain gene-altered ingredients.

TAKING ACTION
AGAINST THE GRAIN

CHAPTER 7

Identifying Your
Sensitivity to Grains

D eciding exactly how far you need to go against the grain for your best health can be confusing because grains can contribute to so many different health complaints in so many different ways. This chapter will sort through the confusion by highlighting the three big grain-related sensitivities—carbohydrate sensitivity, gluten sensitivity, and wheat sensitivity—and will help you assess your risk for each one.

One key point: If you've been eating a lot of refined wheat like most Americans, you're at risk for any of these conditions: carbohydrate sensitivity from too many refined grains and sugars; gluten sensitivity from too much gluten in the diet (perhaps along with other environmental and genetic factors); and sensitivities and allergy-addictions to wheat or other grains that are eaten repeatedly.

What follows is an in-depth look at the main grain-related sensitivities. Based on my experience counseling clients and interviewing researchers and practitioners, I tend to think that there are spectrums of carbohydrate sensitivity, gluten sensitivity, and wheat sensitivity, ranging from very low to very high (see the chart on pages 108–110). Some people are extremely gluten and wheat sensitive but not that carbohydrate sensitive; others are sensitive in all three categories; some have a very strong allergy to wheat but are not gluten sensitive and only moderately carbohydrate sensitive; and so on.

The Three Big Grain-Related Sensitivities

1. Carbohydrate Sensitivity

Caused from an excessive intake of carbohydrates, especially refined wheat and sugars (combined with a lack of nutrients to process them efficiently), sometimes along with genetic factors

The Spectrum of Sensitivity

Healthy blood sugar metabolism

Glucose intolerance
Blood sugar highs and lows, often characterized by
tiredness or irritability after meals and cravings for
quick-fix sweets and refined grain products

Insulin resistance
Difficulty utilizing insulin, often but not always
characterized by weight gain, especially
through the middle of the body

Syndrome X
A more serious form of insulin resistance
characterized by abdominal obesity, high blood
pressure, high cholesterol, and/or high triglycerides

Type 2 diabetes
The most serious form of insulin resistance
characterized by high blood sugar levels and
symptoms such as frequent thirst, frequent urination,
frequent hunger, and fatigue

2. Gluten Sensitivity

Caused from eating gluten, found in wheat and other grains, perhaps along with other environmental factors (stress, viruses, infections, surgery, pregnancy, the use of certain drugs, and the total amount of gluten eaten), and genetic factors

The Spectrum of Sensitivity

Little or no sensitivity

Immune system reactions (gluten sensitivity)
in the gastrointestinal tract
Often characterized by gastrointestinal symptoms such as bloating, but sometimes there are no symptoms

Immune system reactions (gluten sensitivity) in the blood,
which can affect any system of the body
Characterized by symptoms ranging from none to mild to severe, with minor damage and malabsorption in the small intestine sometimes taking place

Silent celiac disease
Characterized by little or no symptoms but with the autoimmune response and overt damage in the small intestine (and often health complications) that characterize celiac disease

Classic celiac disease
Characterized by the autoimmune reaction and severe damage in the small intestine with overt gastrointestinal symptoms and often serious health complications

3. Wheat Sensitivity

Caused from eating too much wheat (pasta, bread, bagels, cookies, and so on), perhaps along with environmental factors and genetic factors

The Spectrum of Sensitivity

Little or no sensitivity
▼
Inflammation and immune system reactions
(wheat sensitivity) in the intestinal tract
Often characterized by minor gastrointestinal symptoms
▼
Immune system reactions (wheat sensitivity)
in the blood that can affect any system of the body
Characterized by symptoms and healthcomplaints
ranging from minor to severe in nature and
sometimes including strong cravings for wheat

To help you get an idea of where you think you rate on the spectrum of these various sensitivities, this chapter has three different symptom/risk factor questionnaires and descriptions of relevant and convenient medical tests. Once you take the quizzes and have additional tests done if desired or if they're indicated, you'll be able to use the information you gain to decide which against-the-grain diet is best for you and, later, to individualize your diet so it's just right for you.

Now that you've seen the range of health problems that can occur within each category, it's time to look at how you fare with each sensitivity individually.

Assessing Your Sensitivity to Carbohydrates

Most of us have eaten refined wheat products and sugar all our lives, so nearly all of us have one degree or another of carbohydrate sensitivity.

The following quiz, while not entirely scientific, should help you learn more about how carbohydrate sensitive you are.

Carbohydrate Sensitivity Quiz

1. Do you eat, or have you had a history of eating (such as since childhood), refined grain products (bread, pasta, bagels, pretzels) and/or sweets every day?
   ___✓___ Yes (4 points)   _____ No (0 points)

2. Do you drink, or have you had a history of drinking, two or more drinks per day of alcohol, soft drinks, and/or fruit juices?
   ___✓___ Yes (4 points)   _____ No (0 points)

3. Do you crave or really love to eat sweets and refined grain products (pasta, bread, baked goods)?
   ___✓___ Yes (4 points)   _____ No (0 points)

4. **a.** Are you ten to twenty pounds overweight and are you carrying it around the middle?
   _____ Yes (7 points)   ___✓___ No (0 points)
   b. Are you more than twenty pounds overweight and are you carrying it around the middle?
   _____ Yes (10 points)   ___✓___ No (0 points)

5. Do you have high blood pressure (consistently above 140/90), or are you taking medication to control your blood pressure?
   _____ Yes (10 points)   ___✓___ No (0 points)

6. Do you have high cholesterol levels (above 240 mg/dl) or a poor HDL cholesterol to LDL cholesterol ratio—or are you taking medication to control your cholesterol?
   _____ Yes (10 points)   ___✓___ No (0 points)

7. Do you have high triglycerides (above 160 mg/dl), or are you taking medication to control your triglycerides?
____ Yes (10 points)   __✓ No (0 points)

8. Do you feel a need to urinate frequently, often experience unexplained thirst, or have prediabetic blood sugar levels (above 114 mg/dl)?
__✓ Yes (10 points)   ____ No (0 points)

9. Have you been diagnosed with either adult-onset diabetes (also known as Type 2 or non-insulin-dependent diabetes) or coronary heart disease?
____ Yes (20 points)   __✓ No (0 points)

10. If you're a woman, have you been diagnosed with polycystic ovary syndrome (PCOS), or do you have irregular menstrual periods, high blood levels of testosterone, excess facial hair, acne, and difficulty getting pregnant?
__✓ Yes (15 points)   ____ No (0 points)

11. If you're a man, do you have premature baldness?
____ Yes (7 points)   ____ No (0 points)

12. Do you have breast, prostate, pancreatic, or colon cancer?
____ Yes (10 points)   __✓ No (0 points)

13. Do you have cognitive disorders, impaired thinking, or dementia?
____ Yes (5 points)   __✓ No (0 points)

14. Do you have a relative or relatives who have or had Type 2 diabetes or coronary heart disease?
__✓ Yes (7 points)   ____ No (0 points)

15. Were you a low-weight baby at birth, or were you ever fifteen pounds or more overweight and carrying it around the waist?
____ Yes (5 points)   __✓ No (0 points)

Total Points __44__

If your points total less than 10, congratulations. You score well in the area of carbohydrate sensitivity and tolerance. You should simply work to maintain that level of health by following a moderate-carbohydrate diet (high in vegetables and low in sugar and refined grains) and keeping a watchful eye out for early signs of carbohydrate intolerance: weight gain, cravings for sweets and refined grain products, and tiredness or irritability after meals.

If your points total 10 to 19, you likely have some level of carbohydrate intolerance, insulin resistance, and high insulin levels, and can be helped by a lower carbohydrate diet that is lower in grains. To get a better indication of exactly how well your body is processing carbohydrates, you might consider asking your doctor to perform a blood test to have your insulin levels measured.

If your points total 20 to 29, you almost certainly have or are at strong risk for insulin resistance and high insulin levels and should follow a lower carbohydrate, grain-free diet to reverse these conditions and stave off your risk of numerous degenerative diseases. To get more information to better assess your health condition, a fasting blood insulin test, and possibly a two-hour postmeal insulin test, is suggested.

If your points total 30 or above, you almost certainly have insulin resistance or Syndrome X and are at strong risk for developing serious health complications, such as heart disease or adult-onset diabetes, if you don't have these conditions already. Blood insulin tests are highly recommended to give you more information about your condition, and it's imperative that you take strong corrective action now by adopting a low-carbohydrate, grain-free diet.

Carbohydrate Sensitivity Tests

To assess a person's blood sugar (glucose) and insulin levels and determine carbohydrate sensitivity and insulin resistance, there are many tests that a doctor can do. One of the most common is the oral glucose tolerance test, in which a patient fasts for some time and then drinks a solution containing 75 grams of glucose or dextrose. Blood is periodically drawn over a two- to five-hour period to determine how high the glucose levels rise and how quickly they fall off. Doctors directly measure changes in glucose and infer insulin function from this data. A glucose response more typical of a diabetic or prediabetic suggests insulin resistance.

A big drawback to this test is that drinking a high-sugar solution can cause extremely uncomfortable symptoms in many people. In addition, the sugar solution that is used is usually made from corn, so abnormal responses may indicate corn sensitivity more than blood sugar abnormalities. To modify the test and make it less stressful and more accurate, patients can eat a breakfast of juice, toast, and cereal (instead of drinking a glucose solution), and then have blood drawn two hours later to measure glucose levels. When the test is conducted this way, it's more patient friendly. Even so, the test still isn't advised for patients who have fasting blood glucose levels above 150 milligrams per deciliter (mg/dl).

The following are the two easiest, least stressful, and most informative tests for assessing how well the body is metabolizing carbohydrates.

Fasting Blood Glucose Test

A fasting blood glucose test is one of a battery of tests routinely done when blood is drawn for standard blood work. Since many people have an annual physical, they can assess their blood glucose levels on a yearly basis to monitor their blood glucose metabolism.

- In general, a normal fasting glucose (taken in the morning, before eating or drinking) should be between 65 and 110 mg/dl.

- An optimal range is between 75 and 90 mg/dl.

Tests for Carbohydrate Sensitivity at a Glance

Oral Glucose Tolerance Test

- Can cause uncomfortable symptoms but can be modified to be less stressful
- Not advised for patients with fasting glucose levels above 150 mg/dl

Fasting Blood Glucose Test

- Provides useful information and is part of standard blood work
- Abnormally high readings usually only appear in the later stages of carbohydrate sensitivity

Fasting Blood Insulin Test

- The best way to assess insulin levels
- Not a common test, so usually needs to be specifically requested by patient

Two-Hour Postprandial Insulin Test or the Insulin Challenge Test

- Provides more in-depth information to determine insulin function and insulin resistance
- Only done by special request or by nutritionally oriented specialists

Low blood glucose levels can indicate hypoglycemia, one of the early signs of carbohydrate sensitivity, and high blood glucose levels can indicate later stages of carbohydrate sensitivity: prediabetes (glucose levels above 114 mg/dl) and diabetes (glucose levels above 126 mg/dl). However, the body pumps out high levels of insulin for a long time to keep blood glucose levels relatively stable, so even if you have a fasting blood glucose reading in the normal range, that doesn't necessarily mean your carbohydrate metabolism is healthy.

Blood Insulin Tests

A fasting blood insulin test is the best way to assess high levels of insulin in the blood, which, as you remember, contributes to many serious health problems. However, this test is not commonly performed in general practice. As awareness of insulin resistance and Syndrome X increases, this test will likely become more commonly used. In the meantime, you can specifically request this test from a general practitioner, or you can opt to see a nutritionally oriented physician or cardiologist who specializes in the treatment of Syndrome X and uses this test routinely.

Many physicians who perform the fasting blood insulin test also perform a two-hour postmeal insulin test or sometimes an insulin challenge test. In the two-hour postmeal insulin test, a patient eats a breakfast—sometimes a typical American Diabetic Association–approved, high-carbohydrate breakfast (cereal, milk, toast, and juice)—and then blood is drawn from the patient two hours later to get a two-hour insulin reading. The doctor can find out how much insulin the body is producing when exposed to a high intake of carbohydrates and will therefore get a much better understanding of how insulin resistant the patient is. The insulin challenge test involves injecting insulin into a blood vessel of the patient and monitoring his or her blood glucose responses every fifteen minutes for two hours. Both tests provide additional information for assessing the severity of insulin resistance.

A healthy fasting insulin level is below 10 micro-international units per milliliter (mcIU/ml), but the lower the number, the better, says insulin expert Ron Rosedale, M.D., of the Colorado Center for Metabolic Medicine in Boulder. He has all his patients have their fasting blood insulin levels measured as part of standard blood work.

Assessing Your Sensitivity to Gluten

Most of us have eaten gluten in the form of wheat all our lives, so virtually all of us have been exposed to the key culprit in this condition. Not all of us have the genes that make us susceptible to developing gluten sensitivity, but genes may not be as important as other environmental factors,

such as stress, viruses, surgery, the use of certain drugs, nutrient deficiencies, and an excessive intake of gluten.

Although most Americans have never heard of gluten sensitivity, it is
very common: celiac disease occurs in at least 1 in every 111 healthy
American adults, and gluten sensitivity may occur in 50 percent or more
of the population. Many people are walking around with gluten sensitivity right now and don't know it. The following quiz can help you get an
indication of whether you might have it.

Gluten Sensitivity/Celiac Disease Quiz

1. Do you eat, or have a history of eating (such as since childhood), a lot
   of wheat or other gluten-containing grains, such as rye, barley, oats, triticale, spelt, or kamut?
   ___✓ Yes (4 points)   ___ No (0 points)

2. Do you either love and crave wheat, or does wheat seem to bother
   you?
   ___✓ Yes (4 points)   ___ No (0 points)

3. Do you feel you have trouble digesting food, or do you have chronic or
   frequent digestive bloating, gas, indigestion, abdominal pain, or an irritable bowel?
   ___✓ Yes (4 points)   ___ No (0 points)

4. Do you have chronic or frequent diarrhea, constipation, nausea, or vom-
   iting?
   ___✓ Yes (4 points)   ___ No (0 points)

5. Do you have dental enamel defects (vertical or horizontal grooves in
   permanent teeth that are often chalky white) or recurring canker sores
   in your mouth?
   ___ Yes (8 points)   ___ No (0 points)

6. Do you have nagging, unexplained chronic fatigue, depression, bone pain, joint aches, or headaches, including migraines?
   ____ Yes (4 points)   ____ No (0 points)

7. Do you have frequent yeast infections that keep coming back after treatment?
   ____ Yes (3 points)   ____ No (0 points)

8. Did many of your unexplained health problems begin following a virus, infection, pregnancy, surgery, or a period of extreme stress?
   ____ Yes (3 points)   ____ No (0 points)

9. Have you ever been diagnosed with unexplained iron deficiency anemia or other nutrient deficiencies?
   ____ Yes (7 points)   ____ No (0 points)

10. Do you have any of the following conditions? (Add 20 points for each condition that you check.)

    ____ Any autoimmune syndrome (such as autoimmune thyroid disease, autoimmune liver disease, or connective tissue disease)

    ____ Arthritis, especially rheumatoid arthritis

    ____ Autism

    ____ Chronic, severe headaches that don't respond to conventional therapies

    ____ Dermatitis herpetiformis (itchy, blistering skin disease)

    ____ Depression that doesn't respond to conventional treatment

    ____ Down's syndrome

    ____ Elevated liver enzymes (SGOT, SGPT, etc.) of unknown origin

    ____ Infertility or a history of miscarriages or pregnancies of poor outcome

    ____ Intestinal cancer, especially T-cell lymphoma or esophageal, pharyngeal, or mouth cancer

_____ Liver disorders of unknown cause

_____ Lupus erythematosus

_____ Neurological disorders of unknown cause, including:

    _____ ataxia (unsteady gait and shaky movements)

    _____ neuropathy (weakness and numbness of the limbs)

    _____ memory impairment

    _____ epilepsy with a history of migraines, chronic gastrointestinal symptoms, attention deficit hyperactivity disease, and/or cerebral calcifications

_____ Osteoporosis or low bone density

_____ Psoriasis

_____ Schizophrenia

_____ Short stature as a child

_____ Sjorgen's syndrome (dry-eye, dry-mouth syndrome, usually with joint inflammation)

_____ Type 1 diabetes

11. Do you have two or more close relatives who have any of the conditions listed in question 10?
    __✓ Yes (10 points)   _____ No (0 points)

12. Do you have a parent who has Type 1 diabetes?
    _____ Yes (15 points)   __✓ No (0 points)

13. Do you have a close relative who has been diagnosed with celiac disease or gluten sensitivity?
    _____ Yes (20 points)   _____ No (0 points)

14. Have you ever been diagnosed with celiac disease or dermatitis herpetiformis?
    _____ Yes (30 points)   __✓ No (0 points)

Total Points _____ 53

If your points total less than 10, gluten sensitivity is likely not a problem for you. Keep in mind that too much gluten can contribute to health problems, even for those who aren't especially sensitive to it, so use this book to learn how to keep your intake low and to become aware of warning signs to watch out for: digestive bloating and gastrointestinal upset; iron or other nutrient deficiencies; and unexplained ill health, such as depression, fatigue, anemia, skin conditions, and reproductive problems.

If your points total 10 to 19, there is a chance you could have gluten sensitivity. A gluten sensitivity test, especially a stool test that detects more minor cases, is helpful for knowing for sure—or simply try a gluten-free diet to see if you feel better eating that way.

If your points total 20 to 29, it's much more likely that you have gluten sensitivity or celiac disease or are at significant risk for these conditions and likely could benefit from a gluten-free diet. It's highly recommended that you have a gluten sensitivity stool test or blood screen done to get more information about the status of your health condition so you can take the appropriate action. This is especially advised if you're a relative of a celiac or if you answered yes to any of the conditions in question 10.

If your points total more than 30, you may very well have celiac disease, or at the very least, you have strong indicators that gluten sensitivity could be contributing to your health problems and should be investigated further. A strict gluten-free diet should be beneficial to you, but it's imperative that you have a blood screen or gluten sensitivity test first to assess how serious your condition is. If you already have celiac disease, you should have periodic gluten sensitivity tests to make sure that your body has healed and that you aren't unknowingly eating gluten, which is hidden in many common foods.

Gluten Sensitivity Tests and Screens

Incredible technological advancements in the area of gluten sensitivity screens have occurred in just the last few years. That's allowed researchers to discover that gluten sensitivity is far more common than anybody ever imagined. It's a lot easier to find out if you're gluten sensitive now than it used to be and it's likely to get even easier in the future. Here are the most important tests to know about for celiac disease and gluten sensitivity—and their advantages and disadvantages.

Intestinal Biopsy

For decades, an intestinal biopsy has been considered the "gold standard" for the diagnosis of celiac disease—in other words, positive results on this test are considered the main criteria for making a celiac disease diagnosis. However, the biopsy has many drawbacks.

Usually an outpatient procedure performed by a gastroenterologist, the biopsy involves inserting a long tube through the mouth and gastrointestinal tract of the patient into the small intestine where several samples of mucosa lining are taken. Then they're analyzed under a microscope. This test obviously is invasive, not to mention expensive. As you might imagine, many patients are reluctant or unwilling to have this procedure done.

Even for those who do have a biopsy done, the test has some inconsistencies. In celiac disease, there isn't universal damage throughout the small intestine—the lesions are patchy—so samples may sometimes be taken from areas that aren't damaged. Biopsies, therefore, sometimes are negative, even though the patient really has celiac disease. In the worst case, accidents sometimes occur in which the intestine is cut and damaged during the biopsy procedure.

In addition, the all-or-nothing approach—the idea that you either have celiac disease or no disease at all—forces millions of people that could be helped by a gluten-free diet to slip through the cracks of the present system. Many people who have normal or near-normal biopsies still

Tests for Gluten Sensitivity and Celiac Disease at a Glance

Intestinal Biopsy

- Specific for determining or ruling out celiac disease
- An invasive procedure in which accidents occasionally occur

Antitissue Transglutaminase (anti-tTG) and Antiendomysial Blood Screens

- Very sensitive and specific blood tests for celiac disease
- More patient friendly because they involve a simple blood test

IgG and IgA Antigliadin Blood Screens

- A simple blood test
- Good for picking up gluten sensitivity in the earlier stages before celiac disease
- A good initial screen for celiac disease

Gluten Sensitivity Stool Test

- The most sensitive test for detecting early stages of gluten sensitivity
- Great for kids and other people who don't want to be stuck with a needle

have gluten sensitivity. Although the intestinal samples of many gluten-sensitive people appear normal under a microscope, up to one-half of these people already have gluten-dependent nutrient malabsorption that is contributing to many forms of ill health and serious health complications such as osteoporosis. To work around the many disadvantages of intestinal biopsies, less invasive, more sensitive screens can be used.

Antigliadin Blood Test

A simple blood test that measures IgA and IgG antibodies to gliadin has long been used as the initial screening test for celiac disease. Gliadin, as you might remember, is the subfraction of gluten that's known to be involved in the celiac disease process. The antigliadin IgA and IgG tests are sensitive but not always specific: in other words, if you have celiac disease, one or both of the tests will pick it up more than 90 percent of the time. However, if you don't have celiac disease, one of the tests may give a false-positive reading.

The antigliadin blood test screens for people who are reacting to gliadin—in other words, it identifies people who have gluten sensitivity. Some people who are gluten sensitive have celiac disease or go on to develop celiac disease later on if they keep eating gluten, and some don't. But even those who don't develop celiac disease have gliadin-dependent symptoms and conditions that can be cleared up by getting gluten out of their diets.

The controversy over the antigliadin blood test is this: many celiac disease specialists want to do away with the antigliadin test because it's not specific enough for celiac disease. However, this is just plain silly from a health consumer's point of view. Although it's helpful for us to know whether or not we have celiac disease, people mainly want to know if they need to remove gluten from their diet for their best health. Anybody who tests positive on the antigliadin blood test is gluten sensitive and should eliminate gluten to improve health and prevent serious health complications.

Blood Tests Specific for Celiac Disease

If one or both of the antigliadin blood tests (IgG and IgA) come back positive, one or both of the following more sophisticated, specific blood screens should be used to determine if the gluten sensitivity has advanced into celiac disease:

- IgA antiendomysial test
- IgA antitissue transglutaminase (anti-tTG) test

The antiendomysial test has been around a little longer (about ten years in Europe and about five years in the United States); the anti-tTG test is the new kid on the block. If you have celiac disease, the antiendomysial test comes up positive nearly 100 percent of the time. If you don't have celiac disease, it comes back negative about 95 percent of the time. The anti-tTG is equivalent in accuracy. Research with these two tests is ongoing, and each test has its advocates. However, it appears the tTG ELISA (which stands for enzyme-linked immunosorbent assay) may win out and replace the antiendomysial test. It may even replace intestinal biopsies as the "gold standard" of diagnosis, which would be a welcome relief for patients. Equally exciting news for consumers is that a skin-prick tTG test taken from a single drop of blood has been developed and should be available to consumers within a year. This will make screening for celiac disease fast, simple, and affordable.

In the meantime, you can ask your doctor to do these tests for you. If your doctor isn't agreeable to this—or if you would prefer not to have the cost of a doctor visit on top of the cost of the test—there are two easy alternatives for having yourself tested:

- If you can't find someone in your area to take your blood, you can contact a consumer-oriented company called Better Health USA (www.betterhealthusa.com). The company can send a technician directly to your home or office to draw your blood and mail your sample to a reliable lab, and the results of your test(s) will be sent directly to you.

- If you can get a medical technician or nurse to draw your blood (probably at the request of your doctor), you can order the antigliadin and anti-tTG tests through a Web site run by a doctor who specializes in gluten sensitivity and food allergies, James Braly, M.D. (www.drbralyallergyrelief.com). All the material you need for the test, along with return mailing packages, will be sent to you, and the results also are mailed directly to you.

More information about these options is in Resources.

Gluten Sensitivity Stool Test

The newest test for gluten sensitivity is a stool test recently developed by gastrointestinal specialist, Kenneth Fine, M.D., of the Intestinal Health Institute. A few years ago he saw that many people who seemed to be intolerant to gluten didn't always have positive antigliadin blood tests, and he suspected that these antibodies should be detected more frequently in the stool of gluten-sensitive individuals than in the blood (because the immune reaction to gluten begins and occurs in the intestinal tract). He conducted research with more than five hundred people and found that to indeed be the case, then decided to bring his innovative test directly to the public via his Web site (www.finerhealth.com) and his lab's Web site (www.enterolab.com) so that people could more easily determine if they have gluten sensitivity.

The gluten sensitivity stool test that he developed can detect antibodies in the stool whether a person has symptoms or not. It's by far the most sensitive gluten sensitivity test available and can therefore pick up cases of gluten sensitivity in the early stages of the disease process before malabsorption and complications develop or become serious. It's a great test for children or adults who don't want to be stuck with a needle. It's also affordable.

To have the test done, you simply have to sign up for the test, wait for a packet of material to be sent to you, give a stool sample in the privacy of your own home, have the sample picked up by an express mail carrier, and wait for the results to be sent to you. See Resources for more information.

The gluten sensitivity stool test and the antigliadin blood screen are two good options for helping to detect gluten sensitivity. The stool test hasn't been used as long, but it's already proven to be more sensitive—it can pick up early immune responses to gluten before gluten sensitivity becomes apparent in the blood.

Assessing Your Sensitivity to Wheat

Except for those who grew up in isolated areas (say, some regions of Africa, or a remote island), all of us have eaten wheat and all of us in the Western world have eaten wheat since a very young age. Not only that, we usually eat wheat several times a day every day. It shouldn't be surprising, therefore, that wheat is one of the top two food sensitivities, right up there with milk. The following quiz, while not entirely scientific, should help you get an idea whether wheat sensitivity is a problem for you.

Wheat Sensitivity Quiz

1. Do you eat some wheat-containing foods (pasta, bread, muffins, cookies, cereal, sandwiches) every day?
   ____ Yes (5 points)　　　____ No (0 points)

2. Do you have digestive bloating and upset, indigestion, or water retention?
   ____ Yes (5 points)　　　____ No (0 points)

3. Do you have frequent diarrhea or constipation?
   ____ Yes (5 points)　　　____ No (0 points)

4. Do you have frequent sinus problems, earaches, or headaches?
   ____ Yes (5 points)　　　____ No (0 points)

5. Do you have allergies, asthma, or frequent rashes?
   ____ Yes (5 points)　　　____ No (0 points)

6. Do you suffer from unexplained hyperactivity, depression, sleepiness after meals, fatigue, and/or joint and muscle aches?
   ____ Yes (5 points)　　　____ No (0 points)

7. Are you overweight even though you don't eat much food except for a few low-fat or fat-free wheat products?
   ____ **Yes (7 points)** ____ **No (0 points)**

8. Do you crave or love to eat wheat-based foods (pasta, bread, pizza, bagels, muffins, pretzels, cookies)?
   ____ **Yes**, often or constantly **(5 points)**
   ____ **Yes**, occasionally **(3 points)**
   ____ **No (0 points)**

9. Do you start eating your favorite wheat-based foods and sometimes feel like you can't stop or feel like you can't get enough of them?
   ____ **Yes (7 points)** ____ **No (0 points)**

10. Do you feel like you can't imagine not having wheat-containing foods (bread, pasta, pizza, pretzels, cookies, cake, pies) in your diet?
    ____ **Yes (5 points)** ____ **No (0 points)**

Total Points _____

If your points total less than 10, wheat sensitivity is probably not a problem for you. It never hurts, though, to have a food sensitivity test or gluten sensitivity test done, or to try a wheat-free diet, just to be sure. You'll learn in the next chapter that emphasizing vegetables in place of wheat products is an excellent strategy for long-term weight control and health, whether or not you're sensitive to wheat.

If your points total 10 to 19, you may have some degree of wheat sensitivity and might benefit from a wheat-free diet or from a food allergy test that screens for wheat sensitivity. Keep in mind that some people who are wheat sensitive are also gluten sensitive, so you should consider having a gluten sensitivity test, too, to catch gluten sensitivity in the early stages before it does a lot of damage.

If your points total more than 20, you may very well have wheat sensitivity, perhaps a strong or long-standing case of it, and you probably will benefit from going on a wheat-free, and possibly gluten-free, diet. You can try either diet to see if you get results. However, before you do, it's highly recommended that you have a wheat sensitivity test and especially a gluten sensitivity test to learn more about your condition, so that you can take the appropriate therapeutic action with your diet and stave off serious health complications.

A special note about corn: Like wheat, corn is a very common food allergen. Many people don't think they eat much corn until they find out all the foods it's in: it's found not just as corn on the cob and sweet corn and in corn tortillas, chips, and most Mexican food (nachos, tacos, taco salads) but also in food products that contain corn syrup, high-fructose corn syrup, cornstarch, and other ingredients. That includes all regular soft drinks and many baked goods and convenience foods.

To give yourself the most thorough assessment concerning your sensitivity to grains, take the Wheat Sensitivity Quiz (see page 126) again, but substitute corn and corn products in place of wheat and wheat products in the questions and see what your score is.

Food Allergy Tests for Detecting Wheat Sensitivity

A number of blood tests to detect sensitivities to wheat, corn, and other foods are available. The IgG ELISA blood test for delayed food allergies seems to be the most accurate, reliable, and reproducible. It involves drawing a single tube of blood and testing it for the presence of IgG antibodies formed against various foods. If your blood shows high levels of IgG antibodies against wheat or other foods, it means you have an immune sensitivity to that food.

Having an IgG ELISA test done often takes the guesswork out of figuring out which foods you're sensitive to, especially if you think you may have multiple food sensitivities. Depending on the lab used, the test usually measures antibody levels to about one hundred different foods. However, the test isn't always accurate. If you have not eaten a food in a while

Tests for Wheat Sensitivity at a Glance

IgG ELISA Food Allergy Test

- Helpful for assessing hidden sensitivities to wheat and a wide variety of other foods at the same time
- A pricey test, but a good investment for people with chronic, unexplained health problems

Wheat Elimination Diet Test

- May be the ultimate test for assessing improvements in health
- Costs nothing

Gluten Sensitivity Test

- Provides information that's useful for preventing future health problems
- A prudent test to have done if you think you're wheat sensitive

or aren't eating enough of it, the test for that food may come out negative, even though you are sensitive to it. In addition, the test can be pricey. However, it's accurate the majority of the time, and it's a good investment for many people who have a lot of allergic symptoms or nagging, unexplainable health problems.

If you can't convince your doctor to do this test for you, you have two options for taking matters into your own hands:

- If you need a technician to be sent to your home or office to draw your blood for you, you can order the test through Better Health USA (www.betterhealthusa.com).

- If you would prefer to do a simple pinprick test of your finger on your own (to get just a drop or two of blood), you can order this test through a company called York Nutritional Laboratories, Inc. (www.yorkallergyusa.com).

More information on these companies is in Resources.

The Food Elimination Diet Test and the Gluten Sensitivity Test

Eliminating wheat or other foods that you think you might be sensitive to and seeing how you feel a few weeks later really is the ultimate test. Anyone can try a wheat-free diet at any time, and most people who do, get unexpected positive results.

However, there is one big drawback to jumping immediately into a wheat-free diet: you may have gluten sensitivity or celiac disease and not know it. More often than not, if you are sensitive to wheat, you're also sensitive to gluten. That means you should be avoiding other grains such as rye and barley as well as numerous food additives. If you eliminate wheat, you may feel dramatically better, but if you don't know you're gluten sensitive, you may continue to eat other forms of gluten that are sabotaging your health. Therefore, if you score high on the Wheat Sensitivity Quiz, it's strongly recommended that you have a gluten sensitivity test performed (either the antigliadin stool test or blood test) to rule out whether you have this insidious condition that can lead to so many serious health complications.

Now that you've learned all about assessing your risk for the three main grain-related sensitivities—and about more tests you might want to have done—you've gained valuable personal information about yourself that will help you determine the best against-the-grain diet for you. In the next chapter, you will learn about nutritional strategies that enhance health and are common to all the against-the-grain diets.

CHAPTER 8

The Against-the-Grain Diet Guidelines

The three different against-the-grain diets are based on the same general concept: replacing some or all of the grains in the diet with vegetables (and, to a lesser extent, other nutritious foods). The main way they differ is the extent to which the diets go against the grain. The Wheat-Free Against-the-Grain Diet eliminates just wheat products. The Gluten-Free Against-the-Grain Diet eliminates wheat as well as other gluten grains (rye, barley, oats, triticale, spelt, and kamut). The Totally Against-the-Grain Diet eliminates all grains. Each diet is covered in detail in Chapters 12 through 14.

No matter how radical my prescription for an against-the-grain diet may seem to you at first, consider that the evidence is overwhelming that eating more vegetables (and to a lesser extent, fruits) protects against degenerative diseases, from heart disease to cancer. No nutritionist who has looked at the medical literature could honestly argue that grains are more important for health than vegetables. (Well, maybe the only exception would be a nutritionist who has been strongly influenced by food manufacturers!)

It's hard to pull ourselves away from the idea that grains are incredibly healthy and necessary for us. It's an idea that has been ingrained into all our psyches since our very early years, but it's a false one. Keep in mind that our earliest ancestors survived very well—thrived, in fact,

The Against-the-Grain Diet Guidelines

1. Reduce or avoid grains and eat more nonstarchy vegetables in their place.

2. Avoid sugar, fructose, high-fructose corn syrup, and other concentrated sweeteners.

3. Enrich your diet with adequate amounts of protein throughout the day.

4. Increase your intake of omega-3 fats and eliminate the bad fats— omega-6-rich vegetable oils and trans-fatty acids.

5. Emphasize monounsaturated fats, such as olive oil, avocados, and nuts, in your diet.

6. Adjust your intake of fruits, starchy vegetables, legumes, alcohol, and dairy products according to your carbohydrate and food sensitivities.

7. Opt for foods in as natural and fresh a state as possible.

unless they had the misfortune of being eaten by a wild animal—without any grains in their diets. We, too, can take grains out of our diets (either completely or partially), eat a large amount of vegetables, as they did, and experience much better health in the process.

Keep in mind that limiting problematic grains is crucial, but eating anything else in sight doesn't necessarily lead to health. As one case in point, celiacs who give up eating gluten sometimes end up eating a lot of high-carbohydrate, gluten-free foods and sweets, and then develop problems associated with carbohydrate sensitivity. So, it's important not to eat one type of junk in place of another type of junk—for example, grain-free sweets that contain bad fats in place of regular sweets with bad fats.

To keep you on track for getting the best sources of carbohydrates, protein, fats, and vitamins and minerals to promote optimal health, I've listed in the sidebar above, seven simple, health-enhancing nutrition principles that are common to all three against-the-grain diets. Now I'll take a closer look at each one.

AGAINST-THE-GRAIN GUIDELINE 1
Reduce or Avoid Grains and
Eat More Nonstarchy Vegetables

The message of this book is that grains have a slew of nutritional problems, and we're not designed to experience optimal health on large amounts of them. Reducing or avoiding grains in the diet, therefore, is key to promoting long-term health and to preventing and reversing minor ailments and serious diseases.

Although limiting grains is a general guideline helpful for everyone, each of us needs to individualize this guideline by determining how far against the grain we personally need to go. Some of us, such as those who don't show any signs of sensitivity to grains but need to lose a few pounds, simply need to greatly limit wheat products. Others, such as those who have celiac disease, a strong sensitivity or allergy to wheat or other grains, or grain addiction, need to completely eliminate even traces of the grains that cause problems, including those found in food additives. (You'll learn more about how to identify hidden sources of grains in convenience foods in Chapter 10.)

Based on how you fared on the questionnaires in the last chapter (and on any follow-up medical tests you have done), you should have a good idea of which against-the-grain diet seems most right for you to begin following. Generally speaking, you should follow the diet for several weeks, and if you get positive results, keep following it and watch your health dramatically improve. If you don't respond as well as you would like to on the diet, don't be afraid to experiment with variations of the diet: avoid other grains (listed in the sidebar on page 134) that may be problematic for you, then reintroduce them and assess how you feel. In most cases, your body will clearly indicate if certain grains deter your health.

Once you limit grains in general and eliminate the grains that are specific problem foods for you, the next question is what will you eat in place

Members of the Grain/Grass Family

The first six grains on the list are gluten grains. They, along with corn, tend to be the most problematic for people. The safety of oats for those with gluten sensitivity is still being debated: it may be safe, but it is almost always processed and stored in the same location as other gluten grains, so it can pick up some gluten through cross-contamination. For that reason, it shouldn't be used by celiacs unless their condition is monitored by a physician.

Wheat, kamut, and spelt	Teff
Triticale (a wheat-rye hybrid)	Millet
Rye and barley	Corn
Oats	Sorghum
Rice and wild rice	Sugarcane and cane sugar

of grains? The simple answer is more vegetables, especially nonstarchy vegetables, such as salad greens, salad vegetables, green beans, and asparagus. Nonstarchy vegetables, as I've explained throughout this book, are the best carbohydrate sources on all fronts: they promote steady blood sugar and insulin levels, are low in carbohydrates, and are rich in fiber, antioxidants, and phytochemicals (plant-based chemicals that protect against disease).

A key idea: By substituting nonstarchy vegetables for grains, you automatically lower the carbohydrate content of your diet, as long as you don't load up on carbohydrate-rich foods, such as sweets, other grains, or potatoes, and continue to eat the same amount or more of other foods, such as meats and fats. Nearly every client who comes to see me eats too many fiber-stripped refined-wheat products and not enough vegetables. So, the number one counseling advice I give in my practice is to switch wheat for veggies. When my clients follow this advice, they experience countless improvements in health, simply from eating a more nutrient-dense diet with fewer carbohydrates. If they're wheat sensitive or moder-

Nonstarchy Vegetables: The Ones to Emphasize

Asparagus	Lettuces and greens
Bok choy	Mushrooms
Broccoli	Spinach
Cauliflower	Sweet and hot pepper
Celery	Yellow wax beans and green beans
Cucumber	
Green, red, and Chinese cabbage	Zucchini and yellow summer squash

ately carbohydrate sensitive (which is common), they experience even more dramatic benefits. This is the strategy on which the Wheat-Free Against-the-Grain Diet is based. The other against-the-grain diets take this basic strategy a bit further.

AGAINST-THE-GRAIN GUIDELINE 2
Avoid Sugar, Fructose, High-Fructose Corn Syrup, and Other Concentrated Sweeteners

Just as the human body isn't designed to handle many grains, it isn't designed to handle many concentrated sweeteners either. Eating a lot of concentrated sweeteners stresses the body's glucose and insulin mechanisms and sets the stage for the development of the most common degenerative conditions that plague North Americans today—excess weight, obesity, Syndrome X, polycystic ovary syndrome, heart disease, Type 2 diabetes, cognitive disorders, and some types of cancer.

Virtually everyone who eats the high-refined-carbohydrate, American diet is carbohydrate sensitive (or prediabetic) to one extent or another because of overeating either sugars or refined grains or both. To prevent and reverse insulin resistance and all the degenerative diseases it is associated with, it's essential to avoid both types of foods, at least most of the time.

Interestingly enough, the most nutrient-poor, highly refined sweeteners are those derived from members of the grain/grass family: sugar, fructose, high-fructose corn syrup, and corn syrup.

If, on occasion, you want to splurge on a nutritious treat, try making goodies using small amounts of fruit, the sweet herb stevia, stevia plus fructooligosaccharides (FOS), or Lo Han fruit juice concentrate, known commercially as Sweet Balance or HerbaSweet. (This low-glycemic sweetener is derived from the Chinese Lo Han fruit, which contains intensely sweet, noncaloric compounds called glycosides.) Other choices that may be appropriate in limited amounts for some people are non-grain-derived glycerin, xylitol, or sucralose. Even small amounts of caloric, natural sweeteners—such as honey, maple syrup, maple sugar, date sugar, or fruit juice concentrate—are okay for special-occasion treats, except for those who are severely insulin resistant. Natural sweeteners have the advantage of being more nutritious than refined sweeteners, but they contribute to blood sugar and insulin spikes, just like sugar, so they shouldn't be overdone. If you're going to cheat on a birthday or special occasion, though, it's far better to use natural sweeteners than refined sweeteners. I'll give you some examples of how to make both grain- or gluten-free and refined sugar-free treats in the dessert recipes in Chapter 15, but think of natural sweeteners as every-once-in-a-while dips into the honeycomb in what otherwise should be a sweetener-free way of life.

AGAINST-THE-GRAIN GUIDELINE 3
Enrich Your Diet with Adequate Amounts of Protein Throughout the Day

The diet our Paleolithic ancestors ate contained between 19 and 35 percent protein. The average American eats a diet with 12 to 15 percent protein. Virtually all of us, therefore, could stand to eat a little more protein for better health; some of us could benefit by eating a lot more.

The word *protein* is derived from the Greek word *proteios*, which means "first" or "of primary importance." This is a fitting term when you realize all of protein's unique functions. Protein is used to build and repair all tissues; make hormones, which regulate body functions; and form

The Quick Way to Identify Refined Sweeteners on Labels

Sugar and sweeteners are found in large amounts in most sweets and are hidden in small amounts in the vast majority of convenience foods. The quick way to identify refined sweeteners on the label is to look for:

- The word *sugar* in any form (such as sugar, cane sugar, brown sugar, or turbinado sugar)
- Words ending in *-ose* (such as fructose, sucrose, or dextrose)
- High-fructose corn syrup, corn syrup, and corn-syrup solids

enzymes, which improve everything from digestion to energy production, maintain the body's fluid and alkaline-acid balance, and make antibodies that are vital for strong immunity. Protein also stimulates the production of glucagon, a hormone that opposes insulin and allows the body to burn stored fat. If you want to lose or maintain weight and have your body functioning in tip-top shape, it is absolutely essential that you consume adequate amounts of protein throughout the day.

Based on my experience with clients, many people give little thought to eating much protein, except maybe at dinner. It's simply impossible, though, to eat the amount of protein that the body needs each day in one sitting. Furthermore, when you eat protein only at one meal, you're eating too many carbohydrates at other meals to keep glucose and insulin levels in healthy ranges—and almost certainly too many refined grain products.

If you really want to control carbohydrate cravings, stimulate weight loss, and improve immunity, digestion, and hormonal function, you need to think of protein as more than a dietary afterthought: instead, protein needs to become a cornerstone of your diet. In other words, eat small amounts of high-quality protein throughout the day, preferably at every meal or snack.

The exact amount of protein you need will vary according to your unique biochemistry. *Three to four ounces of animal protein—about the size of a deck of cards or the palm of your hand—three times a day is a good starting amount for most people.* Those with weakened immunity or those who do strength training may need more protein, and those who are extremely insulin resistant may need less. (Protein can contribute to elevated insulin levels in some individuals, so those with difficult-to-control diabetes may do better with half the standard amount of protein for each meal.) Once again, some individual experimentation is best for determining the ideal amount (and type) of protein for you. The important thing to understand, though, is that no matter who you are, optimal health depends on receiving adequate protein.

Animal foods, such as chicken, turkey, seafood, red meat, game meats, and eggs are all rich sources of protein. They're also the types of protein we are best suited for. The highest quality animal proteins are: meats from animals and fowl that are fed grass, not grain; wild game meats, such as venison, rabbit, and game birds; and eggs from chickens that are fed omega-3-rich flaxseed or fish meal instead of corn. Although not widely available, these protein sources have healthier fatty acid profiles than those of commercially raised animals. Look for them at farmers' markets and health food stores or special order them through the mail or at your local health food store.

The best types of commercial meat are fresh, unprocessed chicken and turkey and lean cuts of lamb, beef, and pork. Organic sources are preferable whenever possible. Processed meat products, such as luncheon meats, are okay in a pinch if other sources of protein aren't available but shouldn't be eaten on a daily basis because of the many additives they contain. Deep-fried meats are unhealthy and should be avoided.

Vegetarians can meet their protein needs through nonmeat sources and still go against the grain, but it's a little harder to do. That's because vegetarian protein sources have nutritional problems that animal foods tend not to have. For example, legumes, like grains, have high amounts of carbohydrates that can be problematic for carbohydrate-sensitive people. In addition, legumes, like grains, are high in antinutrients and lectins, which can promote the development of nutrient deficiencies and autoim-

Protein Sources

Meats
Commercial meat, preferably organic (chicken, turkey, lamb, beef, pork)
Grass-fed animals
Wild game meats (venison, buffalo, rabbit, game birds)

Seafood

Other Animal Sources
Dairy (cheese, milk, yogurt)
Eggs, preferably omega-3 enriched
Whey protein powders
Egg protein powders

Plant Sources
Nuts and nut butters
Seeds
Legumes
Soy foods and soy protein powders
Rice protein powders

mune diseases. Soy, in particular, is a common food allergen and many soy foods contain hidden gluten.

Nuts and seeds offer some protein, often along with significant amounts of beneficial fat, especially monounsaturated fat. Therefore, they can be healthy additions to the diets of both vegetarians and meat-eaters. Other protein options include dairy foods such as cheese, whey protein powders (from milk), soy protein powder, rice protein powder, and egg protein powder. Because most of the foods from which these products are derived are relatively new foods in our diet, the healthfulness of these foods needs to be evaluated on an individual basis.

Vegetarians should experiment with protein sources and decide which ones are best for them. In some cases, if vegetarians have food sensitivities to key protein sources, such as soy foods and dairy products, they may need to add omega-3-enriched eggs and omega-3-rich fish to their diet to receive adequate protein and beneficial fats.

AGAINST-THE-GRAIN GUIDELINE 4
Increase Your Intake of Omega-3 Fats and Eliminate the Bad Fats—Omega-6 Oils and Trans-Fats

Another key to health is balancing the good fats in your diet and eliminating the bad. One type of fat we need for health, omega-3 fatty acids, is found primarily in cold-water fish, and the other type, omega-6 fatty acids, is found in small amounts in most plant foods and in high amounts in vegetable oils, such as corn oil, soybean oil, cottonseed oil, peanut oil, safflower oil, and sunflower oil. Omega-3 and omega-6 essential fatty acids (EFAs) work in opposing ways in the body, and both are very good when they're in balance. However, when omega-6s are in excess—as they are in the typical American diet—they become bad.

That's because omega-6s produce hormonelike substances that promote inflammation, whereas omega-3s produce hormonelike substances that are anti-inflammatory. Excess omega-6s also have been found to promote insulin resistance and obesity, not to mention the growth of some cancers. Omega-3s, on the other hand, help improve insulin sensitivity and retard the growth of some cancers.

A greatly overlooked issue regarding fat, therefore, is balancing out the two different types of EFAs in the unbalanced American diet. Americans currently eat ten to twenty times more omega-6s than omega-3s, whereas the ideal ratio is between 1:1 and 4:1. Too little omega-3 fatty acids contributes to many health problems because the body needs omega-3 fatty acids to produce flexible cell membranes, which in turn help insulin work properly.

The main way to correct the all-important EFA balance in the body is to completely eliminate omega-6 vegetable oils (and reduce your intake of grains) at the same time that you increase your intake of both omega-3

Five Important Ways to Boost Your Intake of Omega-3 Fats

1. Eat more cold-water fish, such as salmon, trout, tuna, sardines, herring, and anchovies. It's best to eat these fish three times a week, but eating them just once a week helps reduce your risk of heart attack.

2. Add raw flaxseed oil to salad dressings and on top of cooked foods. Or sprinkle flaxseeds on salads or cereals (such as gluten-free muesli) or use in baked goods or protein bars or shakes.

3. Use omega-3-enriched eggs from chickens fed fish meal or flaxseeds. Also look for meat and milk from animals that are fed these omega-3-rich foods, for grass-fed meats, and for game meats, such as venison, buffalo, and game birds.

4. Eat a lot of dark green, leafy vegetables. Good sources of omega-3 EFAs are romaine lettuce, mesclun mixed greens, arugula, kale, and collard and mustard greens.

5. If you don't like fatty fish or the food ideas above—or if you need high amounts of omega-3s to try to counter excess inflammation in the body or insulin resistance—your best bet might be to take fish-oil supplements that contain omega-3 fats (with vitamin E to prevent rancidity).

fatty acids and monounsaturated fats. Monounsaturated fats will be covered in the next guideline.

In addition to eliminating omega-6-rich vegetable oils, it's of equal importance to eliminate the other bad fats—trans-fatty acids, which are found in margarine, vegetable shortening, deep-fried foods, and foods that contain partially hydrogenated oils. Trans-fatty acids are shaped differently than the polyunsaturated fatty acids from which they are made, so they act like molecular misfits in the body, adversely affecting crucial cell membrane and EFA functions. Research shows that trans-fatty acids: raise total cholesterol; lower "good" HDL cholesterol; increase "bad" LDL cholesterol; raise lipoprotein (a); and promote blood platelet stickiness, each a strong risk factor for heart disease. Furthermore, diets high in trans-fatty acids promote insulin resistance and Syndrome X and double the risk of heart disease. These fats offer no nutritional benefits but plenty of health risks, so you should do everything in your power to avoid them.

AGAINST-THE-GRAIN GUIDELINE 5
Emphasize Monounsaturated Fats in Your Diet

Unlike omega-3 fatty acids, monounsaturated fats aren't essential to health—the body can manufacture monounsaturated fatty acids from other fats, protein, or carbohydrate if it needs to. Nevertheless, emphasizing monounsaturated fats in the diet is healthful, especially when you reduce your carbohydrate and grain intake. Sources of monounsaturated fats include olives, olive oil, almonds, hazelnuts (and hazelnut oil), cashews, pistachios (and pistachio oil), pecans, macadamia nuts, and avocados.

Monounsaturated fats offer many benefits. First, they are flavorful, satisfying additions to the diet that don't raise insulin levels and are fantastic for balancing blood sugar levels. Second, substituting monounsaturated fats for carbohydrates improves insulin sensitivity. Eating more monounsaturated fats and omega-3 fats, therefore, is very effective medicine for anyone with carbohydrate sensitivity, including diabetics and those with Syndrome X. Third, monounsaturated fats increase levels of the good HDL cholesterol, help reduce total or LDL cholesterol levels, and inhibit the oxidation of LDL cholesterol. (Oxidized LDL cholesterol is more likely to set the stage for heart disease than regular LDL cholesterol.) Fourth, more monounsaturated fats in the diet may reduce the risk of breast cancer.

An easy way to eat more monounsaturated fats is to use unrefined or cold-pressed extra virgin olive oil as your primary oil in place of omega-

Sources of Monounsaturated Fats

Almonds	Macadamia nuts
Avocados	Olives and olive oil
Cashews	Pecans
Hazelnuts and hazelnut oil	Pistachios and pistachio oil

6-rich vegetable oils in salads and cooking. Olive oil is particularly healthful because it has mild antithrombotic (anticlotting) properties. If you would like a little variety, hazelnut or pistachio oils can also be used—both monounsaturated-rich oils offer unique flavor to dishes, especially to salad dressings.

Also, use avocados in meals, and snack on nuts, such as hazelnuts and almonds, instead of pretzels or popcorn. All these monounsaturated fat sources have been found to lower cholesterol levels. They are also rich in heart-healthy nutrients such as vitamin E. Numerous studies have found that eating nuts significantly lowers the risk of coronary heart disease. One caveat to keep in mind, though: if you have an allergy or sensitivity to one or more nuts, do not eat them. No matter how healthy nuts may be, they are not healthy for *you* if your body allergically reacts to them.

AGAINST-THE-GRAIN GUIDELINE 6
Adjust Your Intake of Fruits, Starchy Vegetables, Legumes, Dairy Products, and Alcohol According to Your Sensitivities

The diet should be based on the three essentials that made up our original diet—high-quality protein, nonstarchy vegetables, and good fats. A diet that supplies only these food groups meets all our nutritional needs and is extremely therapeutic (as well as preventive) for a wide variety of conditions. If you have serious health problems, such as diabetes or an autoimmune disease, you need to stick pretty close to these original food groups alone for your best nutritional chance of recovering your health.

The rest of us can usually add other types of other foods—such as fruits, starchy vegetables, legumes, dairy products, and small amounts of alcohol—for more variety in our diets. However, the amounts and types of these foods that each of us should include in the diet is really a matter of individual biochemistry and how carbohydrate sensitive and immunologically sensitive we are.

Fruits and Starchy Vegetables

Generally speaking, most of us should favor—in this order—nonstarchy vegetables, fruits, and starchy vegetables (such as yams, sweet potatoes, beets, and winter squash) over legumes and grains. In virtually every study of chronic disease, the higher the consumption of fruits and vegetables, the lower the risk of disease. Although fruits and starchy vegetables aren't as beneficial as low-carbohydrate, nonstarchy vegetables, they still offer protection and are preferable to legumes and grains.

Vegetables and fruits have another big benefit: they are alkaline foods, unlike legumes and grains, which are acidic foods. When the diet is overly acidic, the body pulls calcium out of the bones to buffer the acidity. Therefore, to protect bone health, it's always better to eat vegetables or fruits with meats, poultry, fish, dairy products, and nuts (and even legumes and grains) than to eat, for example, legumes and meats together, which are both acidic.

As beneficial as fruits and starchy vegetables are, most people can only enjoy these foods in small or moderate amounts. If you eat more of these foods than your body can tolerate, you can gain weight or develop high blood cholesterol and triglycerides or other health problems. Therefore, if you are moderately carbohydrate sensitive, add these nutritious foods to your diet, but control your intake and watch how your body responds. The best fruits to try are low-carbohydrate, low-glycemic ones such as berries, plums, nectarines, peaches, and small apples, and the best tolerated starchy vegetables are usually spaghetti squash and unsweetened yams or sweet potatoes.

A Simplified Look at
Acidic and Alkaline Foods[1]

After digestion and absorption, all foods produce either an acid or alkaline load. To promote calcium balance and better bone health, always try to balance acidic foods with alkaline foods in meals.

Acidic (from most acidic to least acidic)
Hard cheeses and processed cheese
Processed meats, such as canned meats and luncheon meats
Whole grains
Fresh meats (red meat and poultry), fish, and eggs
Nuts, refined grains, soft cheese, legumes, yogurt, butter

Neutral
Olive oil

Alkaline (from least alkaline to most alkaline)
All fruits
All vegetables

Legumes

Legumes—beans and peas—rank low to moderate on the glycemic index. That means the carbohydrates they contain are converted to blood sugar slowly, and they therefore produce favorable, low to moderate rises in blood sugar. This is a big plus of legumes.

However, legumes are relatively new foods in the human diet, and, as such, they have many of the same nutritional problems that grains have. As already mentioned, legumes are acidic. They also are high in carbohydrates, so it's easy to overeat them and gain weight. In addition, legumes have a high content of antinutrients and lectins, which increase the risk of developing nutrient deficiencies, gastrointestinal upset, and/or autoimmune disorders. In my clinical experience, most people don't digest legumes well and experience a great deal of gas and bloating from eating them. (I think the same phenomenon might occur from eating grains if most of us ate whole grains. However, since most of us eat refined grains, the adverse effects aren't quite so noticeable.) For all these reasons, it's best to evaluate your tolerance for beans, just as you do grains. If you seem to do well with legumes, control the portions you eat and vary your intake.

Dairy Products

At first glance, dairy foods seem beneficial to health, but like grains, they're not all they're cracked up to be. As you might remember, dairy foods were only introduced into our diet about 10,000 years ago, and we haven't had enough time to adapt and experience our best health on these foods.

Many people eat dairy products because they think milk is good for their bones, but that's a highly debatable point. Keep in mind that our early ancestors and many nonindustrialized societies ate no dairy foods and had stronger bones than most societies who eat dairy foods, including our own.

Although they're rich in calcium, dairy products as a group are acidic and therefore upset calcium balance in the body. Cheeses, especially hard cheeses, are the *most* acidic foods. So, using cheese as a protein source, as many lacto-vegetarians do, is worse for calcium balance and bone health than eating meat. This is especially true if you eat cheese with other acidic foods, such as whole grains and legumes.

Many people also are intolerant to lactose (the sugar in milk), and others don't tolerate certain proteins in milk, such as casein. Gas, bloating, and intestinal upset are just as common from eating milk products as from eating wheat or beans. In addition, cow's milk allergy is the number one food sensitivity, contributing not only to gastrointestinal distress of many types, but also to many cases of asthma, autism, bronchitis, eczema, and increased infections, such as middle-ear infections in children. Furthermore, dairy products contain opioids that set the stage for dairy cravings and addictions in some people, and recent research suggests that the casein in milk may promote insulin resistance in some people.

The evidence indicates that you should be careful with dairy foods and evaluate your sensitivity to them, just as you should with grains. But

Controlling Carbohydrates

If you're mildly carbohydrate sensitive, it's best to limit yourself to no more than a total of five servings of fruits, starchy vegetables, legumes, and tolerated grains. Of all these foods, emphasize fruits; try to limit yourself to three servings per day or less from starches; and favor starchy vegetables and legumes over grains whenever possible.

Serving sizes for fruits are:

1 cup berries (any type)

2 small plums

1 medium peach or nectarine

1 small or ½ medium apple, orange, or pear

1 kiwi

¼ melon (such as cantaloupe or honeydew)

½ cup pineapple

½ banana

Serving sizes for starches are:

1 medium sweet potato or yam

1 cup baked spaghetti squash

1 small or ½ large baked potato

1 cup carrots

½ cup beans, peas, or lentils

½ cup corn

1 slice whole-grain bread

½ cup oatmeal or ½ cup other cooked whole grains

all dairy foods are not bad for everyone, just as all grains aren't bad for everyone. If you seem to do fine with dairy foods, opt for organic sources (free of growth hormones), try to find dairy foods from grass-fed cows, eat dairy foods more as condiments than as staples of your diet, and be sure to eat them with alkaline vegetables or fruits.

If you think you might be sensitive to milk, eliminate all dairy foods for a while, then try some butter and see how you do with it. Butter has little of the problematic proteins in milk that can cause allergies, so it tends to be one of the best tolerated dairy foods.

Alcohol

Alcohol in general should be avoided, especially if you are carbohydrate sensitive. Like refined sugar, most types of alcohol provide empty calories—in other words, calories with no nutritional value. Alcohol also contributes to nutrient deficiencies because it interferes with the absorption of essential nutrients and accelerates their excretion from the body—and it contributes to the development of a leaky gut. In addition, alcohol provides 7 calories per gram (slightly fewer calories than fat does), so it's next to impossible to lose weight when you drink much alcohol.

The liver has to detoxify alcohol (like it does all other drugs), and doing this often disrupts efficient functioning of the liver. Regular use of alcohol, therefore, can lead to sluggish liver function, which in turn can contribute to blood sugar problems, elevated blood cholesterol, food allergies, chemical hypersensitivities, skin problems, hormonal imbalances, and poor elimination.

On the positive side, alcohol relaxes people and often encourages desirable social interactions—two qualities that are compatible with good health. Red wine and, to a lesser extent, white wine and dark beer also have polyphenols, plant chemicals that have antioxidant effects, which may offer some protection against heart disease. However, vegetables and fruits are the richest sources of polyphenols, and most of us can benefit far more by eating more vegetables and fruits (and practicing stress-reduction techniques) than by drinking more wine and beer.

If you want to drink occasionally, opt for wine, drink moderately, and keep the carbohydrate content of your diet extra low on the day you're drinking. That means avoiding grainy snacks and eating only protein and nonstarchy vegetables. This is the most savvy way to enjoy the beneficial effects of alcohol without as many adverse health consequences as usually come with it.

I strongly urge you to avoid hard-distilled liquors, which have no nutritional benefits. Most of these are derived from grain: bourbon (at least half from corn), rye (from rye), scotch (from barley), vodka (from wheat, rye, corn, or potatoes), and rum (from cane products). I also urge you to avoid beer. Although beer contains some nutrients, it also contains gluten, which can contribute to gluten sensitivity, a common condition that can lead to many serious health complications.

AGAINST-THE-GRAIN GUIDELINE 7
Opt for Foods in As Natural and Fresh a State As Possible

Our original diet consisted entirely of fresh, natural, unprocessed foods. The more we can eat unprocessed foods instead of processed foods, the healthier we will tend to be.

There are several reasons why a more natural diet is best. The more a carbohydrate is processed in manufacturing, the higher your body's glucose and insulin responses will be to that food. Remember that the higher your body's glucose and insulin responses, the more energy problems you will tend to have and the more you will set yourself up for long-term glucose- and insulin-related health problems, such as diabetes and heart disease.

This means that whole grains (whichever ones you tolerate) are better for blood sugar than cracked whole grains, and cracked whole grains are better than refined grain products. Similarly, fresh-cooked beans are better than instant beans made out of flakes; an apple is better than applesauce (which in turn is better than apple juice); and fresh vegetables, cooked or raw, are better than canned vegetables. The more you can eat foods in whole-food form, with all their nutrients and fiber intact, the more you will be protected against insulin-related degenerative diseases. (Yes, it's true that whole grains and beans will have more antinutrients than their processed counterparts, but if you react adversely to whole grains and beans, you shouldn't be eating processed forms of those foods either.)

A diet consisting mostly of natural foods also encourages a healthy potassium-to-sodium ratio more similar to the ratio humans evolved on. Virtually all natural foods have a high potassium-to-sodium ratio—in other words, large amounts of potassium and small amounts of sodium. By contrast, when foods are processed and preserved, they lose potassium and gain sodium, and develop a poor potassium-to-sodium ratio. A poor potassium-to-sodium ratio in the diet disrupts normal cell function and increases the risk of high blood pressure, cardiovascular disease, stroke, and cancer. Eating mostly natural foods corrects the ratio and helps prevent degenerative diseases.

When you emphasize unprocessed foods over processed foods, you also automatically steer clear of a wide array of chemical preservatives and additives that are hidden in processed foods. As I explained in Chapter 3, food manufacturers add additives usually for manufacturing reasons, but additives pose real or potential dangers to our health, especially when they're in combination with each other. Some additives in common use now will probably be found unsafe and banned in the future, and many additives are derived from problematic grains and provoke adverse symptoms in those who are sensitive to grains. So, the best defense for protecting yourself (and your family) against both the allergenic and not-yet-recognized, toxic effects of many additives is to eat foods in as natural and unprocessed a state as possible.

Putting the Guidelines into Practice

As you've learned, there are compelling nutritional reasons to follow the against-the-grain eating guidelines. Baffling health problems improve and people feel and look better.

The rest of this book is devoted to helping you apply this information in your life, starting with the next chapter, which psychologically and practically prepares you for the brave, new world of eating against the grain.

CHAPTER 9

Preparing for the Challenges of Going Against the Grain

E ating against the grain isn't easy, especially in the beginning. Physically, your body may crave grains. Emotionally, you may feel a deep sense of loss from giving up foods to which you are attached. Socially, friends and strangers alike will try to coax you into eating grains because "everyone else does." And advertising, marketing, the media, and the government keep subtly pushing you to eat grains at what seems like every turn.

The constant pressure of pro-grain forces can weigh on you and make you feel like you have to go to Herculean efforts to avoid grains. Admittedly, dealing with these forces can be a challenge, but it doesn't have to be impossible. There are some tricks of the trade to make it easier to go down the road less traveled to health and better well-being.

Embrace Change

Most of us have trouble with change, even if it's something we really want. We often cling to old ways of doing things out of habit, inertia, wanting to fit in, or simply because that's the only way we've ever learned. It is the same with our diet. We've eaten grains all our lives, but it's time to be honest with ourselves and realize that eating so many grains isn't working. There simply is no way to rebuild and maintain optimal health without eating against the grain—and you're going to have to rock the boat a little to do that.

Instead of dreading going against the grain, think of it as a golden opportunity to use the latest scientific knowledge to give you a healthy edge. Realize that the high-grain diet most North Americans eat isn't something you should want to emulate. Take the steps that are needed to prepare for this dietary change and look forward to it, then embrace it with open arms.

Fortify Yourself with Knowledge and Incentive

The first step is to understand the health benefits of a low- to no-grain diet. By reading this book, you're well on your way toward that goal. I suggest you reread sections of the book often as a way to counter all the pro-grain hype in our culture with some solid scientific evidence and sound reasoning. The best offense against pro-grain pressure is a good defense of knowledge.

What you've read so far should provide the incentive you need to begin eating against the grain. To stick with an against-the-grain diet, keep fortifying yourself with this information. Try writing down important passages from the book on Post-It notes and place them on your computer, desk, or refrigerator. Check out Web sites or read other books that give you additional information or invest in a subscription to *Sully's Living Without*, a magazine that is all about people who are creatively coping in the real world without gluten grains and other hard-to-avoid foods.

Do What's Right for You

All of us like to fit in to one extent or another, but fitting in isn't worth the price of long-term poor health. Without health, little else matters. Have the courage to eat what's best for you, even if that means being a little different and politely but firmly speaking up for what you need. With the increasing popularity of protein-rich diets these days, it's a lot easier to follow a no- or low-grain diet without feeling like a total outcast. But if you have trouble letting others know what you need for your best health, consider taking an assertiveness course or joining a celiac support group to build up this skill.

Be prepared that when you don't follow the pack, your friends and acquaintances may get so uncomfortable that they will put heavy-duty pressure on you to eat what they're eating. (Deep down they probably know they're eating junk and know they should avoid it, just like you are.) Don't let their pressure deter you from following your path to health, but don't try to push your way of living on them either. Simply adopt a "live and let live" attitude and realize that sharing positive experiences with people who care about you is more important than being a conformist who eats the same food.

As a woman who was raised to be a people pleaser, I know this isn't always easy. My best suggestion, though, is to stop trying to be like everyone else and to slowly but surely become comfortable with your own uniqueness. With grain sensitivity or anything else, the more you learn to accept yourself (and become open about many different aspects of yourself), the more others tend to sense it and like you for the real you. If you have the courage to do what's best for you, you often find other people, much to your surprise, will end up following your example.

Deal with Your Feelings

It's amazing how something so simple as changing your diet can conjure up so many different feelings, but it does. First, there might be relief and excitement because you've found the answer to your health problems. But, that's usually followed by lots of other feelings, such as sorrow (for giving up foods you have fond memories of), resentment (because eating against the grain isn't as convenient as eating the grain-based foods everyone else does), and anger and disappointment (because your friends and loved ones aren't as understanding and supportive about this dietary change as you would like them to be).

If you experience these emotions, don't think there's something wrong with you. Conflicted feelings are a natural part of dealing with the loss that comes with change. Accept the feelings, be compassionate about them, and take time to work through them. But also keep in mind the reason you're making the change: to experience health improvements you haven't been able to experience any other way.

Look for emotional support from friends and family members. If they aren't very supportive, use this experience as an opportunity to learn to communicate better with them. Tell them how difficult this change is and how important it is for you to have their support even if they don't understand exactly why you have to eat this way. Be sure to reinforce positive behavior by thanking them when they're thoughtful of your needs.

Another way to seek out emotional (and practical) support is to join a gluten-free, low-carb or food allergy support group or an Internet chat group. If you do better with one-on-one advice, consider hiring a nutrition counselor who can offer solutions to your particular needs.

Learn New, Practical Skills

Learning new, practical skills to replace old eating and food-preparation habits is a crucial part of following an against-the-grain diet. Then you need to practice those skills over and over until they become second nature.

The next two chapters will guide you through the nitty-gritty details of how to grocery shop and eat out against the grain. Here, though, are some general guidelines for following any of the against-the-grain diets at home.

1. **Plan ahead.**
    This is rule number 1 for eating against the grain. You can't grab any grain-based convenience food on the spur of the moment without sabotaging your health, so you have to give a bit more thought to what you're going to eat. Then prepare accordingly. Have ready-to-eat vegetables and fruits on hand at home. Get into the habit of carrying nuts and other healthy foods for you to eat. Keep your refrigerator and freezer well stocked with protein-rich eggs, poultry, lean meats,

and fish, and set aside enough time in your schedule to prepare these foods.

2. **Eat enough protein.**
    This is guideline number 3 in the previous chapter, but it bears repeating. If you have strong cravings for grains and sugars, it's very likely that you're not eating enough protein, especially for breakfast (see guideline 7 on page 156). Along with avoiding the grains that provoke cravings, eating enough protein is the most common dietary solution for controlling cravings. If that isn't the answer, try eating more good fats, such as olive oil, nuts, and fatty fish.

3. **Keep sweets and problematic grains out of your house and always have substitute foods on hand.**
    The easiest way not to cheat is not to have ready access to problematic foods. Prepare for the urge for quick, between-meal snacks by stocking healthy, ready-to-eat, grain-free, sugar-free foods, such as hard-boiled eggs, cooked meats, cans of low-sodium tuna, veggie sticks, and fruits.

    Also, look for healthier substitutes for problematic, grain-based, convenience foods. For example, if you're gluten sensitive but not particularly carbohydrate sensitive, use gluten-free breads, waffles, and pasta on occasion to replace the foods you may be missing.

    Using gluten-free substitutes is a great technique for transitioning over to a gluten-free diet, but it's important not to overeat these foods. No matter which diet you follow, you should always make a conscious effort to eat more vegetables and fruits than grains.

4. **Keep meal preparation simple.**
    When you eat against the grain the right way, food preparation becomes much less involved. The meals, in turn, become much more healing. Steer away from complicated recipes that contain a dozen or more ingredients and delight in simplicity. By using just a few fresh or seasonal foods and no processed foods, easy, uncomplicated dishes take on a gourmet taste. For example, sprinkling a dried herb between the skin and flesh of a chicken breast and placing it in the oven

doesn't take a lot of time, but the end result is extremely tasty. By steaming up a big serving of vegetables, you have yourself a meal.

5. **Purposely make leftovers.**
    If you make more food than you plan to eat in one sitting, you have pre-prepared food to snack on or to use as an ingredient in quick meals later in the week. This tried-but-true technique makes it much easier to follow the against-the-grain diet and usually helps save money, too.

6. **Look for shortcuts to healthy meal preparation.**
    Have the meat counter clerk cut meat up for you for quick stir-fries or kabobs, and buy prepackaged, prewashed salad mixes or veggie sticks. These are important survival strategies for getting through the times when you are just beginning the against-the-grain diet, are under a lot of stress, or feel too tired to cook meals from scratch.

7. **Be creative, resourceful, and original about eating foods that are good for you.**
    To eat against the grain, it's important to break out of the bonds of traditional meals and get creative. For example, many of my grain-sensitive clients feel better eating lunch or dinner foods—say, leftover chicken or steak, vegetables, and brown rice—for breakfast. This may initially sound a bit strange, but eating dinner for breakfast really is a nutritious way to start the day.

One client of mine often has fish for breakfast. This wouldn't be my breakfast of choice, but it works for her and that's all that matters. Other off-the-beaten-path ideas include poached eggs on hash brown potatoes or poached eggs on sautéed vegetable medleys. Many celiacs I know get in the habit of carrying veggie sticks or acceptable crackers to parties where they know they can eat the dips.

We all have a tendency to get into ruts with the foods we eat, but there are lots of different, tasty, grain-free foods out there. Put your thinking cap on and be original. You might just start a trend!

Take the Diet Challenge

If you're overwhelmed by the whole against-the-grain idea, take things one step at a time and do what you can. As a short experiment, try one of these challenges:

- *The best test:* Try the against-the-grain diet that seems best for you for just two weeks.

- *A second option:* If you don't think you can follow the diet for two weeks, make the commitment to try it for one week only.

- *A third option:* If you don't think you can follow the grain-free or gluten-free diet for one week, try the wheat-free diet for one week instead.

It really is a small sacrifice to try a new diet for seven days, particularly if you've been plagued by health problems that haven't improved no matter what type of therapy you've tried. What do you have to lose? Understand that the change may be hard for the first several days, but anyone can try something for a week. Simply take it one day at a time.

At the end of the week, evaluate how you feel. If you feel worse, you can stop the diet if you want to. But if you feel better, keep following the diet. Never think about where this experiment will lead or how long it will go. Just keep taking it one day at a time and let the symptoms your body gives you guide you.

Be Patient with Yourself and the Time Needed to Change

None of us are ever perfect with our diets, especially when we're making the transition from our old way of eating to our new way of eating. We're only human, grains are everywhere, and the pressure to eat grains is strong.

Actually, after following a short against-the-grain diet challenge, trying a small amount of a grain you've avoided is one way you learn what you shouldn't eat. (Having said that, though, I must emphasize that people with celiac disease, especially silent celiac disease, can't afford to experiment with gluten grains.) If you experience a strong reaction from eating a grain you haven't eaten in a while, the chances are good that you're not going to want to experience that reaction again.

Changing long-standing habits is an up-and-down process, though. It may take several negative experiences to convince you to steer clear of problematic grains. It's important to be patient and forgiving with yourself. Realize that dietary mistakes are a natural part of learning, and over the long haul, nothing is a more powerful teacher and promoter of change than personal experience.

Whenever you fall off the anti-grain wagon, don't get discouraged and give up. Just pick yourself up and get back on. Psychologists who specialize in encouraging long-term change say we should be prepared for backslides when we're under stress. This is part of being human. The people who successfully adapt to change persevere and don't let momentary slip-ups deter them.

So, don't dwell on dietary transgressions. Laugh them off and learn from them. The more you keep going back on the against-the-grain diet, the more it will become a comfortable way of living from which you will not want to stray.

CHAPTER 10

Shopping
Against the Grain

A re you ready to build up your practical skills for steering clear of grains in the real world? In this chapter, you'll learn the ins and outs of grocery shopping against the grain. In the next chapter, you'll learn all about eating out against the grain.

Supermarket savvy is covered first because selecting tasty, grain-free foods at the store allows you to eat and cook against the grain at home. It's also helpful for another reason: the more you read food labels, the more you get an idea of the many foods where traces of grains may be lurking. This knowledge can help you navigate around problem foods in restaurants or wherever you may go.

Grocery Shopping 101

There's a knack to shopping against the grain—whether in grocery stores or natural food stores—and it involves one simple guideline: *Avoid the inner aisles and shop mostly on the outer edges.*

Supermarket design is relatively consistent from store to store. The freshest, healthiest, and most grain-free foods—vegetables, fruits, meat, seafood, frozen foods, eggs, and dairy foods—are on the perimeter of supermarkets.

Convenience foods with long shelf lives, by contrast, line the inner aisles of all stores. The vast majority of these foods are made out of grains (especially refined flour), and often sweeteners, processed fats, and additives. That means they're precisely the products you want to avoid.

Shopping against the grain requires breaking old habits and may seem strange at first, but it is by far the best way to shop. When you learn to pick up mainly produce, meat, and seafood, your shopping experience becomes simpler, faster, and often cheaper.

Shopping Basics at the Grocery Store

The following is a quick guide of the ingredients to watch out for—and the foods you should emphasize—on a trip to the supermarket. Wheat, gluten, and corn are hidden in countless commercial products, so your best bet is to focus on fresh, unprocessed foods (those that have no label at all).

"Veg Out": The Produce Section

One of the key guidelines of against-the-grain eating is to emphasize a wide variety of fresh vegetables and, to a lesser extent, fruits. That means you should spend much, if not most, of your time shopping in the produce department.

Nonstarchy vegetables (those that aren't root vegetables or winter squash) and fresh herbs should form the bulk of the produce you buy. If you're extremely carbohydrate sensitive, they should be the only produce you buy.

If you are not very carbohydrate sensitive and don't need to lose weight, you can afford to experiment with virtually any fruit and vegetable: just be sure to keep portions of carbohydrate-dense vegetables and fruits, such as potatoes, tropical fruits, and dried fruits, moderate. If you start to gain weight or have cravings from eating these foods, that's a clear sign that you need to reduce your intake or avoid them and stick solely to nonstarchy vegetables.

One more important point regarding produce: try to buy organic varieties whenever possible. Buying organic protects you from the pesticides, fungicides, and other chemicals that are often used on commercial produce. But it's also the best bet for avoiding unlabeled, genetically engineered vegetables and fruits, which can contain chemicals, lectins, or other allergenic substances.

If your local grocery store doesn't carry organic produce, look in other stores or your local natural food store, or try farmers' markets. If you cannot buy organic, peel your fruits and vegetables, or use a fruit and vegetable rinse that contains a food-grade nonionic surfactant, such as OrganiClean (1-888-VEG-WASH), a product that can usually be found in health food stores.

Meaty Matters: The Meat and Seafood Sections

You should also regularly visit the meat and seafood departments of the supermarket. Rule number 1 is to choose items that are as fresh and unprocessed as possible. The following are tips for making gluten-free selections in these departments.

- Select fresh, unprocessed meats or poultry over those that are pre-basted, deep basted, premarinated, smoked, and cured, or made into sausage.

- Avoid breaded or floured chicken, turkey, or fish. Breaded foods obviously contain wheat, but many of us overlook these wheat sources.

- Buy fresh fish and seafood instead of processed forms, such as fish cakes, crab cakes, and smoked fish. Choose fish that looks good and smells good and was delivered to the store the most recently.

- If you buy beef in supermarkets, select the leanest cuts you can. Good choices include ground round, flank steak, London broil, eye of the round, and eye-of-the-round breakfast steaks. Remember that commercial beef comes from cattle fattened on grains and has an unhealthy fatty-acid profile, so selecting lean cuts is important. (Meats from grass-fed animals or animals fed omega-3-rich mash are far better choices, but they're difficult to find.)

- If you are very corn sensitive, you may need to seek out grass-fed meats, poultry, and dairy products. These products are sometimes available at farmers' markets. You can also special order them at some health food stores or through the mail. (See Resources.)

A Special Word of Caution

The products that are recommended in this chapter are based on the most current, generally agreed-upon information about the foods and additives that are safe for people with celiac disease and grain sensitivities and those that aren't. However, *you should use this information at your discretion.* Consider that:

- Scientific knowledge of ingredients that provoke food sensitivities continues to be debated and to evolve and change.

- Companies sometimes modify ingredients in their products. (That means it's important to always read labels carefully!)

- No matter what the current research shows or what ingredients are listed on the label, we're all individuals who react differently to various foods and additives.

If there's a suggested product in this chapter that you know you adversely react to—or if you try a new product and experience unpleasant symptoms—by all means avoid it. It's up to you to listen to the signals your body gives you and fine-tune the shopping list guidelines in this chapter so they're personalized for you.

The Cold Shoulder:
The Refrigerated and Frozen Foods Sections

When shopping against the grain, you might also make a quick stop in the refrigerated section of supermarkets. Eggs, a great source of protein, should be number one on your shopping list from this area.

If you've been fearful of the cholesterol in eggs, don't be: the cholesterol they contain has little or no effect on blood cholesterol levels. Furthermore, most supermarkets now offer superior kinds of eggs—

omega-3-enriched eggs from chickens fed omega-3-rich fish meal or flax meal. As you learned in Chapter 9, eating omega-3-enriched eggs is an easy way to increase your intake of omega-3 fats, and eating more omega-3s reduces inflammation and improves insulin sensitivity. Many brands of omega-3-enriched eggs exist, including Gold Circle Farms, Born 3, Eggland's Best, and Pilgrim's Pride's EggPlus.

If you aren't sensitive to dairy, you can pick up butter, nonfat or low-fat cottage cheese, or unsweetened yogurt, or cheeses such as mozzarella and feta. However, it's healthier to buy organic dairy foods, which are free of growth hormones, at natural food stores.

The frozen foods section of the supermarket offers a few helpful products, but it is also packed with many refined grain-based foods. To navigate around the grains, walk past the frozen pizzas, waffles, TV dinners, pasta helpers, and pies and head to the most helpful group of foods in the freezer: the frozen vegetables. Be sure to choose those vegetables with no added seasonings or sauces.

Fresh vegetables are tastier and more nutritious, but frozen vegetables last a lot longer and are ready to cook at a moment's notice. In addition, frozen vegetables often are offered in interesting combinations that you might not be able to find fresh. So, it's always a good idea to buy several different types of frozen vegetables and have them in your freezer. This helps you eat against the grain when you're out of fresh vegetables or just too busy or tired to chop them.

Flash-frozen fish, frozen shrimp, frozen meats, and unsweetened frozen fruits are other healthful, grain-free products that are often available in the frozen case. Always read the list of ingredients on packages carefully and make sure these products contain no additives or hidden ingredients.

Quick Stops in the Inner Aisles

The inner aisles of the supermarket aren't places you should spend much time in, but that doesn't mean you need to avoid them altogether. The following are some of the healthiest choices you might want on your shopping list, as well as a few important reminders of what to avoid.

Beverages

Bottled water, sparkling mineral water, or sparkling water with flavor essences should be priorities on your shopping list (unless you have a water filter at home). Water is the only drink that is a nutrient all by itself; we should drink it often to keep the body in tip-top shape. If the cost of bottled water at your supermarkets is too pricey, try buying it at discount specialty stores such as Trader Joe's or discount warehouses such as Costco.

Steer clear of fruit juices, fruit drinks, and soft drinks sweetened with high-fructose corn syrup and sugar, which have a lot of carbohydrates and little or no fiber. This is one of the easiest things you can do to protect yourself and your kids against carbohydrate sensitivity.

Herbal Teas, Teas, and Coffee

Select plain, unflavored tea, green tea, or coffee to avoid hidden problematic ingredients. Tea, especially green tea, is a better choice than coffee: it is rich in antioxidant compounds and can lower glucose and triglyceride levels. The flavonoids in tea also have been shown to positively influence bone mineral density.

If you're gluten sensitive, don't be tempted to use coffee substitutes in place of coffee. Commercial coffee substitutes contain gluten, usually in the form of rye, barley, or barley malt. The only coffee substitute I know of that does not contain gluten is Herbal Cafe by Nutricology. You can special order this through your health food store or call the company, listed in Resources, directly.

Herbal tea is a flavorful way to drink more water, but it's important to be savvy about the types you choose. Read labels carefully and be sure to avoid varieties that contain malt or barley malt. Also, if "natural flavors" or "artificial flavors" are listed on the ingredients, the tea might contain gluten. You will have to call the company that makes the product to determine if the product is gluten free. If you have celiac disease, the general rule is: *When in doubt, find out (from the company) or leave it out.*

Nuts

As you learned in Chapter 9, nuts are nutritious foods that protect against heart disease, and they make convenient snack foods and entrée toppers. For the best freshness, I recommend purchasing nuts from health food stores that keep nuts refrigerated. However, you also can find raw nuts without additives in the baking aisle of your local supermarket.

Canned Foods

It's best to choose fresh or frozen meats and vegetables over canned, but a few types of canned foods can be on your shopping list. For example, water chestnuts, which typically only come canned, are nice additions to stir fries. Hearts of palm, which taste a lot like artichoke hearts, are good in salads and shrimp, chicken, and spinach sautés. Sliced beets are packed with nutrients, but most people don't have the patience to cook them from scratch. Choosing canned versions of these vegetables, therefore, is a handy way to get more vegetables into your diet.

When you buy canned foods, try to buy the lowest sodium products available. If you can't find low-salt varieties, empty the contents of the can into a strainer and run water over the food: this technique sends much of the excess sodium down the drain.

Canned tuna is another helpful canned food, but gluten can sometimes be hidden in unidentified broths on ingredient lists. StarKist, though, is one safe choice: its entire line of canned tuna is gluten free. The vegetable broth StarKist uses may contain beans and tomatoes: if you're sensitive to these foods, try its Gourmet Choice or low-sodium varieties.

Seasonings

Herbs and spices provide a lot of flavor and phytonutrients with every shake of the bottle, so they are important ingredients to purchase and have on hand at home. To make healthy, safe choices, keep in mind these basics:

- All single dried herbs and most herbal combinations are gluten free.
- Seasoning blends and herbal combinations sometimes contain

monosodium glutamate, hydrolyzed vegetable protein, textured vegetable protein, natural flavors, or other questionable ingredients, so read labels carefully.

- Wheat flour or corn-based fillers are sometimes added to ground spices, such as curry, and not listed on the label. This happens most often in commercial brands. To be sure ground spices don't contain gluten or corn, call the company and ask—or choose ground spices from health food brands such as Frontier Herbs, The Spice Hunter, or Wild Oats private label.

- If you are a celiac, it's okay to buy commercial vanilla and other flavorings extracted with grain-based alcohol, according to new guidelines by the American Dietetic Association. In the opinion of chemists, gluten peptides do not make it through the distillation process. However, if you react adversely to alcohol flavoring extracts—or if you simply want to avoid alcohol—opt for flavorings extracted with non-grain-based glycerin, such as those by Frontier Herbs.

Condiments

Distilled white vinegar or grain vinegar (made from gluten grains or corn) has long been on the no-no list for celiacs, but according to new American Dietetic guidelines, grain vinegar is safe for celiacs, just as alcohol is. That means condiments made with white vinegar, such as capers, olives, salad dressings, and horseradish, should be okay, too.

However, some people (whether celiac or not) adversely react to grain vinegar but not to other vinegars. Therefore, pay attention to how you feel after eating foods made with grain vinegar, and steer clear of these foods if they seem to be problematic for you.

Generally speaking, I think it's best to use wine vinegar, balsamic vinegar, apple cider vinegar, or rice vinegar instead of white vinegar in salad dressings and recipes whenever possible. While the new guidelines might mean many people don't need to be strict about avoiding every drop of grain vinegar hidden in some foods, nongrain vinegars are the better choice. They seem to be better tolerated, they definitely don't have gluten, and they have a lot more flavor than grain vinegar.

The Most Common Sources of Wheat, Gluten, and Corn

Wheat Sources

All foods that contain flour, bread flour, enriched flour, bleached flour, unbleached flour, semolina flour, whole wheat flour—basically any type of flour unless it's labeled 100 percent flour from a different type of grain

Blue cheese and roquefort cheese (wheat is often used in the production of molds)

Bread (except those labeled wheat free), including croutons, pita bread, flour tortillas, nan bread, pizza, chapatis, and some papadums

Breaded entrées, such as fried fish and onion rings

Many breakfast cereals and breakfast bars

Communion wafers

Cookies, cakes, rolls, crackers, muffins, bagels, pancakes, and waffles

Couscous, bulgur wheat, and tabouli

Pasta, including spaghetti, macaroni, egg noodles, shells, bows, vermicelli, and so on

Sauces, soups, bouillons, and gravies made with flour or hydrolyzed vegetable protein

Most soy sauces, shoyu sauces, tamari sauces, teriyaki sauces, and many marinades

Wheat Food Additives

Look out for the following ingredients on content lists; these are often derived from wheat:

Cereal, such as cereal binder, cereal filler, cereal protein, or cereal starch

Starch, such as edible starch, food starch, and modified food starch

Protein of an unspecified source, such as hydrolyzed plant protein (HPP), hydrolyzed vegetable protein (HVP), and textured vegetable protein (TVP)

Caramel color or flavoring, monosodium glutamate (MSG), dextrin, and some artificial flavors (you need to check with companies on the source)

Vanilla and alcohol-distilled flavoring extracts and distilled white vinegar (these are sometimes made from wheat grain distillations and may be safe for most wheat sensitive people, but problematic for others)

Gluten Sources

All the foods and additives listed under wheat plus the following:

Barley malt found in some foods, teas, and other drinks, such as Postum

Beer, ale, and grain alcohols, such as rye, whiskey, bourbon, and scotch

Breads, pasta, cereals, cookies, cakes, and other foods made out of wheat, rye, barley, oats, triticale, spelt, or kamut

Seitan (wheat-gluten-based "meat")

Some seasoning salts or blends or fajita seasoning mixes

Soy meat substitutes that contain vital wheat gluten or soy sauce

Gluten Food Additives

Look out for the following ingredients:

Malt, such as malt, barley malt, malt vinegar, or malt syrup

Mono- and diglycerides, natural flavors, and vegetable gum (these may not contain gluten, but you need to check with companies on their sources for these ingredients)

Brown rice syrup, used to sweeten rice and soy beverages and foods (check with the manufacturer and make sure that barley enzymes are not used in the production process)

Ground spices (wheat flour is sometimes used to prevent clumping)

Corn Sources

Corn on the cob and sweet corn

Cornbread

Cornflakes, corn grits, Cheerios, Corn Pops, and some other breakfast cereals

Corn oil and margarines that contain corn oil

Corn tortillas, corn chips, corn tortilla chips, and some packaged snacks, such as Doritos

Countless convenience foods that contain high-fructose corn syrup, such as crackers, cookies, cereals, sweets, and frozen TV dinners

Gravies, soups, and sauces thickened with cornmeal or cornstarch

Hominy

Polenta

Soft drinks, fruit drinks, and shakes made with high-fructose corn syrup

Corn Food Additives

Look out for the following that are derived, or can be derived, from corn:

Corn, such as cornmeal, cornstarch, corn gluten, corn syrup, and high-fructose corn syrup

Dextrose, glucose syrup, and maltodextrin

Lecithin

MSG

Starch, protein, or vegetable additives, such as cereal starch, vegetable protein, or vegetable oil (you must check with companies on their sources for these ingredients)

Citric acid, which can be derived from wheat or corn; in the United States, it is made from corn, but like grain vinegar and alcohol, it is not believed to cause reactions in most sensitive people

---

Going the Extra Mile:
Shopping in Natural Food Stores

I recommend shopping in natural food supermarkets because they offer more options and healthier alternatives to the products found in grocery stores. First, they carry a wide selection of organic products—foods not sprayed with pesticides; products and produce much less likely to be genetically modified; and meats, eggs, and dairy products from animals not treated with hormones or antibiotics. Natural food stores also offer "cleaner" convenience foods with fewer additives and many wheat-free, gluten-free, and grain-free alternatives. Avoiding food allergens and chemicals is a cardinal rule for promoting health, so going the extra mile to shop in a natural food store makes good sense. (About the only food not readily offered in most health food stores is grass-fed meats. I hope this situation changes because grass-fed meats have less fat, fewer calories, and more beneficial omega-3 fatty acids and beta-carotene than grain-fed meats. They also carry a lower risk of harmful E. coli bacteria.)

Despite the better alternatives in natural food stores, there are a lot of high-carbohydrate, nutrient-poor products, too. For example, baked goods made with white rice flour, potato starch, cornstarch, and tapioca starch may be gluten free, but they provoke blood sugar and insulin spikes and promote nutrient deficiencies just like white flour and sugar do. Sugar-rich sweets can be organic, but that doesn't mean they're healthy: they still promote carbohydrate sensitivity and nutrient deficiencies over the long term. Some products labeled "organic," "all natural," and "gluten free" may be good choices, but others are not.

To make the healthiest choices, become a savvy shopper and look beneath the surface: read labels carefully, watch out for troublesome ingredients, and look at the grams of carbohydrates and sugars per serving. The lower the number of carbohydrates and sugars, the better the product protects against carbohydrate sensitivity.

To keep shopping easy for you, I've created a quick summary of the most helpful food items found in natural food stores. Those that can be used by people on a low-carbohydrate diet are marked with an asterisk (*).

Beverages*

Natural food supermarkets and specialty stores, such as Trader Joe's, often offer imported sparkling mineral waters that are good sources of calcium, in addition to standard brands. All mineral waters quench the body's thirst for water, but mineral waters that offer 5 percent or more of the daily value of calcium (brands such as Mendocino, San Pellegrino, or Gerolsteiner) offer a little extra nutrition for the money. They are especially good choices if you are concerned about getting enough calcium and want to avoid dairy. Research has shown that drinking just one glass of a high-calcium mineral water a day significantly slows calcium loss and therefore protects bone health.

Teas*

Natural food stores usually offer organic types of tea and coffee, as well as a larger selection of green teas, herbal teas, and medicinal teas. Single-herb teas, such as chamomile, peppermint, or ginger, are always good choices: besides being gluten free, they often settle the stomach like nothing else does.

With flavored teas, check with the company to make sure there is no hidden gluten that could deter your recovery if you have celiac disease or gluten sensitivity. A few choices I recommend are any Celestial Seasonings tea that does not list roasted barley or barley malt in the ingredients and any Good Earth tea. (According to these companies, the natural flavors they use are gluten free.)

If you're sensitive to caffeine or want to avoid caffeine in the evening, try one of a couple types of Good Earth green tea, which are decaffeinated by a natural process to preserve the tea's antioxidants. Seelect Herb Ruby Burst red bush tea, available in three flavors, is another antioxidant-rich choice I like. Unlike black tea, green tea, and orange pekoe, red bush tea has tealike flavor without any caffeine.

Broth* and Soups

Broth adds a lot of flavor to vegetable, poultry, fish, and meat dishes, so it should be a regular item on your shopping list. Most commercial brands sold in grocery stores should be avoided because they often contain gluten or corn. Even if they don't, they contain a lot of other unhealthy ingredients—sugar, monosodium glutamate, a wide range of additives and preservatives, unhealthy amounts of salt, and sometimes partially hydrogenated oil.

Fortunately, there are many superior varieties of broth in natural food stores that are suitable for wheat-free, gluten-free, and grain-free diets. Good choices include: Pacific Foods chicken, vegetable, beef, or mushroom broths; Shelton's chicken broth; and Health Valley chicken and beef broth in cans. (Be careful, though: Health Valley's chicken broth and vegetable broth in boxes contains barley malt and, therefore, contains gluten.)

Pacific Foods, Shelton's, and Health Valley make many varieties of soups that are gluten free, as well: just check the ingredients. If you do okay with beans from time to time and aren't carbohydrate sensitive, a nice product to try for a change of pace is Shelton's chicken or turkey chili with beans.

Pasta Sauces

Just like broth, the pasta sauces sold in natural food stores tend to be free of added sugars and preservatives—and gluten. Millina's Finest and Muir Glen Organic Pasta Sauces are two good choices. Trader Joe's also has a number of pasta sauces under its private label that fit the bill. Remember that you don't always have to serve these sauces with pasta: they taste great on meatballs, sautéed julienne vegetables, or baked spaghetti squash.

Salad Dressings*

I recommend homemade salad dressing made with a high-quality oil over commercial salad dressings, which contain refined oils. Homemade dressing doesn't take long to make—one example is tossing greens with olive oil and balsamic vinegar to taste—and it always tastes better than commercial brands. If you want to pick up a dressing for convenience, try:

- Annie's and Wild Oats brand salad dressings: many varieties are made with nongrain vinegar. Add fresh lemon juice for extra flavor. If you're carbohydrate sensitive, avoid varieties that have added sweeteners.
- Zeus Greek Salad Dressing, which is found in some specialty markets.
- Spectrum Omega-3 Vinaigrettes, which contain 2 grams of beneficial omega-3 fats per serving. Using this dressing is a convenient way to get more omega-3s into your diet, but the dressing is sweetened with fruit juice concentrate and is not a good choice if you are carbohydrate sensitive.

Condiments

In the condiment aisle, there are countless products made with grain vinegar (which many gluten-sensitive people say are okay and others say aren't). If you would rather avoid these, look for alternatives made with nongrain vinegars, such as Eden Stone Ground Mustard (made with apple cider vinegar); Westbrae Unsweetened Un-Ketchup (made with apple cider vinegar); Westbrae Catsup (made with apple cider vinegar); and Muir Glen Organic Tomato Ketchup (made with white wine vinegar). The first two are better choices because they aren't sweetened.

Olives are a great monounsaturated-fat-rich snack or low-carbohydrate ingredient to use in salads or Mediterranean recipes. Look for brands made with red wine or white wine vinegar instead of white vinegar and those that don't contain ferrous gluconate (an unnecessary source of added iron used for coloring).

Most tamari and soy sauces—and sauces made with them, such as teriyaki and stir-fry sauces—contain wheat and therefore gluten. Brands that are clearly labeled wheat free, such as one variety by San-J, do not. Some people have trouble with wheat-free tamari, though, so use this product—or Bragg's Liquid Aminos, a soy sauce substitute—at your discretion.

If you have an autoimmune disorder or yeast overgrowth, you may need to avoid foods made with yeast or mold, such as vinegar, alcohol, and cheese. Vinegar-free condiments include: Eden Organic Reduced-Sodium Sauerkraut; Santa Barbara Olive Co. pitted olives; Martinis Pitted Kalamata Olives; and cheese-free pesto sauces such as those by Rising Sun Farms.

Unrefined Sea Salt* and Natural Sweeteners

Regular table salt is gluten free, but it isn't good for health for other reasons: it is refined to remove all naturally occurring minerals besides sodium and chloride, it's bleached and treated with anticaking agents, and it typically contains aluminum and sugar. It's best to bypass table salt as much as possible and buy an unrefined salt to use at home. Real Salt, an unrefined rock salt found in most health food stores, is the brand I most often recommend.

Natural sweeteners, such as stevia, fructoligosaccharides (FOS) and Lo Han fruit sweetener, are used in some of the recipes later in this book. You usually can find these—and calorie-dense, special-occasion sweeteners, such as honey, maple sugar, maple syrup, all-fruit spreads, and fruit juice concentrates—in natural food stores. If you have trouble finding these products, ask your store to special order them or order them through the mail from Omega Nutrition or Allergy Resources (see Resources).

Oils*

Olive oil should be a staple in your kitchen, and natural food stores offer a far wider selection of olive oils than grocery stores. Seek out cold-pressed or unrefined extra-virgin olive oil. *Extra-virgin* is important: it means the oil comes from the first pressing of the olives. Many good brands of extra-virgin olive oil are imported from Greece, Spain, and Italy.

Another occasional addition to your shopping cart might be unre-fined sesame or peanut oil for use in stir-fries. Most all other types of oils—namely, vegetable oils—are refined and high in omega-6 fats and should be avoided. Two exceptions are unrefined hazelnut oil and pista-chio oil. Rich in monounsaturated fats, they're nutty, gourmet treats you can use in salad dressings, on top of cooked vegetables, or in special baked goods. Many health food stores don't carry these oils, but you can order them directly from Omega Nutrition (see Resources).

Coconut Butter*

Another helpful fat to include on your shopping list is, believe it or not, coconut butter (also called coconut oil). A source of saturated fat that does not contribute to heart disease, coconut butter is good to use when making baked goods. Coconut butter whips up easily, has a neutral fla-vor, and is better than butter for greasing cake pans and cookie sheets.

Coconut butter, a very stable fat, is also your best choice for high-temperature cooking. It's far better to cook with coconut butter than to heat omega-6 vegetable oils to high temperatures (and, in the process, create health-damaging free radicals and trans-fatty acids).

With easy-to-digest, medium-chain fatty acids that have antiviral properties, coconut butter is an especially good choice for people who have trouble digesting fat or who have suppressed immune systems. It's also great for people who want a grain-free, dairy-free alternative to but-ter or margarine. The best source for unrefined coconut butter is Omega Nutrition.

Coconut Milk*

Thai Kitchen coconut milk is another handy dairy-free, gluten-free product. You can use the lite variety in place of milk in almost all recipes. The full-fat version is delicious on top of chopped pineapple, papaya, or nectarines for a quick, healthy dessert. If it's not sweet enough for you, just add a touch of pineapple juice.

Nut Butters* and Nuts*

Natural food stores offer a wide variety of unsweetened, unsalted nut butters and raw or plain roasted nuts. If you're sensitive to one type of nut, try another. Choose from almonds, Brazil nuts, cashews, hazelnuts, macadamia nuts, pecans, pistachios, and walnuts, and vary your intake for better nutrition. Almond butter, cashew butter, and hazelnut butter are nice alternatives to peanut butter, and usually better tolerated.

If you have celiac disease or a severe allergy to grains, buy prepackaged nuts rather than nuts in the bulk-foods section to avoid the risk of cross-contamination with gluten or other grains. Trader Joe's offers packaged nuts at good prices.

Keep in mind that if you grind raw nuts, they make nice flours for gluten-free baked goods. Nuts also can be toasted at home for better flavor than that of commercial roasted nuts. To do this, place raw nuts on a shallow cookie sheet and toast at 300 degrees Fahrenheit until warm and fragrant but not burned (about five minutes or so for sliced almonds and ten minutes or so for pecan halves). These tasty morsels are satisfying snacks and wonderful toppers on salads, hot cereals, or steamed vegetables.

Pumpkorn*

Pumpkorn, a snack food sold in health food stores, is another product you might want on your shopping list. Kids like Pumpkorn because it's a "fun" food, but it's also nutritious. It's made from seasoned dry-roasted pumpkin seeds, a good source of protein, healthy fats, and zinc, a mineral that helps insulin function more efficiently. Pumpkorn comes in seven varieties that are all considered wheat and gluten free. Many flavors, such as the original flavor, are made with wheat-free tamari sauce and are low in carbohydrates. If you would rather avoid the tamari and aren't carbohydrate sensitive, try the maple-vanilla flavor.

Flaxseeds,* Flaxseed Oil,* and Flaxseed Meal*

Flaxseed products are regular items that can be found in natural food stores. Flaxseeds are tiny brown or golden seeds rich in omega-3 fatty acids, and flaxseed oil and flaxseed meal are derived from flaxseeds. Each product can be used on top of salads and cooked cereals or vegetables as a way to increase your intake of beneficial omega-3 fats. I prefer the seeds and the meal to the oil and recommend flaxseed meal as a healthful addition to homemade protein bars and breakfast smoothies.

Canned Fish*

Another way to increase your intake of omega-3 fats is to add more fatty fish to your diet. Using canned fish is one convenient way to do that. Unfortunately, manufacturers sometimes dust fish (especially salmon) with flour to prevent it from sticking during the manufacturing process, so traces of gluten can be hidden in canned fish without appearing on the label. If you have celiac disease, you'll have to call the manufacturer of your favorite canned fish to check on its safety.

Another option is to look for canned fish by Crown Prince: it does not dust its fish with flour. Sold exclusively in health food stores, Crown Prince products include tuna, salmon, clams, shrimp, crab meat, oysters, sardines, kipper (herring) snacks, and anchovies. Except for a few products with flour in sauces, all products are free of gluten, corn, dairy, and preservatives.

Frozen Fish Products

In the frozen foods section of the store, you can find Omega Foods salmon burgers and tuna burgers and Northwest Natural halibut burgers, salmon burgers, and tuna with pesto medallions. All these products are gluten free and can be cooked quickly for fast food at its best. Serve them with steamed vegetables or a salad for an easy meal.

Northwest Natural fish products are combined with a wild rice blend—in other words, they're moderate in carbohydrates and not recommended if you are carbohydrate sensitive. Omega Foods burgers, in contrast, are low in carbohydrates. They're appropriate for any of the against-the-grain diets.

Chicken Burgers*

Casual Gourmet chicken burgers and chicken sausages are also in the frozen foods section of many natural food stores. These handy products are gluten free and low in carbohydrates and they're made with antibiotic-, hormone-, and nitrite-free chicken. All these pluses make Casual Gourmet products healthy choices for fast food for most Americans. Their only drawback is they are a bit high in sodium. (To balance out their sodium content, be sure to eat them with lots of vegetables.) If you can't find these products in your local natural food store, you can always ask the store manager to order them for you.

Game Meats and Convenience Meats*

Game meats, such as buffalo, venison, and ostrich, are especially healthy offerings in many natural food stores. They are more expensive than commercial meats, but they have healthier fatty-acid profiles than grain-fed meats. If you can afford them, at least on occasion, include them on your shopping list. They'll add both variety and extra nutrition to your diet.

Fresh meats and poultry should be chosen over processed types most of the time, but there are a few lines of convenience meat products that can fit into a wheat-free, gluten-free, and low-carbohydrate lifestyle. One choice is Shelton's, which makes many gluten-free products, such as turkey sausage, turkey burgers, turkey and chicken franks, and turkey breakfast strips (an alternative to bacon). You can find most of these products in the frozen foods section.

In the deli area of your natural foods supermarket, look for Applegate Farms brand. If it's not there, request its products by name. Applegate Farms offers a line of antibiotic-, steroid-, and growth-hormone-free deli meats that are free of gluten, nitrites, and preservatives—and most items are sugar free.

If You Have Celiac Disease or Gluten Sensitivity . . .

It's important to understand that certain aspects of the gluten-free diet are universally agreed upon and others aren't. European countries have a set of recommendations that differ from other countries, such as the United States, Canada, and Australia. Within the United States, two of the three major celiac support groups agree on a set of eating guidelines; the other one disagrees.

The controversy over the diet surrounds gluten-free grains, some additives distilled from gluten grains, and highly purified wheat starch products. Here is a quick review of those issues:

- Rice, corn, millet, sorghum, and teff are members of the grain family. Amaranth, buckwheat, and quinoa are not truly grains, but they can be used like grains. None of these foods contain gluten, so most celiac authorities say these grains are safe. However, it's possible that lectins or other antinutrients in these foods provoke adverse reactions in some people. Another possibility is that some of these products may be processed in facilities where gluten grains are and may pick up trace amounts of gluten that are bothersome to those who are very sensitive.

- Oats have been found to be safe for celiacs in a few recent studies, but oats are almost always stored and processed in the United States in facilities where gluten grains are. That means there's a high probability of cross-contamination. Some doctors allow oats, but all U.S. celiac organizations recommend against their use. The safest course is not to eat oats unless you have your doctor's approval and regular supervision and monitoring of your condition.

- Alcohol and grain vinegar are often distilled from gluten grains, but scientists believe that gluten doesn't make it through the distillation process. Some people, though, react to these ingredients. This may happen because these people are sensitive to yeast or because alcohol contributes to increased intestinal permeability, which increases allergic reactions.

- European countries allow highly purified wheat-starch food products that contain trace amounts of gluten in them, but studies show that celiacs experience more adverse symptoms when they include these foods in their diet than when they don't. U.S. celiac organizations recommend avoiding these products, and I agree. Even if the trace amounts of gluten in wheat-starch products aren't problematic (and I think they are), these products are nutritionally lifeless foods.

Part of the reason for the controversy surrounding the gluten-free diet is that gluten sensitivity is not a black-and-white, all-or-nothing issue. I believe there are a spectrum of reactions to gluten and grains in general: some people are more sensitive to miniscule amounts than others. Until more research is done, it's best to rely on your own reactions and senses to determine your tolerance for gluten-free grains and additives—what I call the "gray" areas of the gluten-free diet.

Fortunately, there is no disagreement over the foods that are emphasized in the against-the-grain diets. Fish, poultry, meat, vegetables, fruits, and nuts are definitely gluten free and should always form the basis of your diet.

Frozen Vegetables and Fruits

Many companies offer frozen vegetables and fruits, but Cascadian Farms, a health food brand, offers a few helpful foods in its widespread line that other companies don't. One is butternut squash. You can quickly heat up this product, then dress it up with butter or flaxseed oil, cinnamon or pumpkin pie spice, and toasted, chopped pecans. It's a tasty, fiber-rich, gluten-free brunch accompaniment to turkey sausage patties, and it's particularly nice on a cool fall or winter morning.

Another product I wholeheartedly recommend is Cascadian Farms' (pitted) Dark Sweet Cherries. To make one of the easiest desserts possible, put some in a bowl and allow them to thaw for fifteen to thirty minutes.

Soy Foods

Soy foods have been touted as health foods, but they're anything but that for many people. As a group, soy foods actually are one of the most common sources of hidden gluten.

Seitan and most soy-based veggie burgers and meat substitutes (such as Tofurky and others) contain "vital wheat gluten"—the secret ingredient that gives the products the texture and taste of meat. Other common sources of gluten in soy products include textured vegetable protein, hydrolyzed vegetable protein, soy sauce, tamari, monosodium glutamate, and barley malt. Celiacs and gluten- and wheat-sensitive people should avoid these products at all costs—and most other people should as well because these products are loaded with additives that aren't conducive to health. Generally speaking, traditionally prepared soy foods, such as tofu, steamed soy pods, and some types of tempeh and miso, are free of gluten and offer the best health benefits. Be sure to read labels carefully, though. Some types of tempeh and miso contain grains or tamari.

The health hype surrounding soy centers on the phytoestrogens it contains, which play a role in modulating hormonal activity, and the protein in it, which has been found to help lower blood cholesterol levels. Many foods emphasized in the against-the-grain diets offer similar health benefits. Avocados, olive oil, nuts, and garlic have all been found to lower cholesterol levels, just like soy. In addition, all plant foods contain phytoestrogens. If you eat a lot of vegetables and fruits, you will get a lot of natural phytoestrogens in your diet, even if you don't eat soy.

Keep in mind that soy foods frequently provoke digestive bloating, flatulence, and food sensitivities. This is understandable because they contain many of the same antinutrients (such as phytate and lectins) that grains do. It's best to judge your individual tolerance to soy foods, and if you tolerate them, choose high-quality products and avoid eating them over and over again.

Grain Products and Substitutes

Just about anything that's made from wheat (for example, waffles, pasta, and cookies) can be made from other grains, too—and natural food stores offer lots of alternatives. These products come in handy from time to time and can be great substitutes when you're transitioning over to an against-the-grain diet.

However, I cannot emphasize enough that wheat-free products are high in carbohydrates and often contain antinutrients that aggravate gastrointestinal and immune function. These products can be eaten moderately or sparingly if you aren't carbohydrate sensitive, but they shouldn't be eaten repetitively or in large amounts.

The following is a list of wheat-free alternatives that I and some of my clients use. Most are gluten free; those are marked with GF. Always pay attention to your body's reactions to these foods and don't eat any that seem to bother you.

Hot Breakfast Cereals

Ancient Harvest Quinoa Flakes (GF)

Arrowhead Mills Amaranth (GF)

Arrowhead Mills Rice and Shine (cream of rice cereal) (GF)

Arrowhead Mills cream of rye or cream of barley or any variety of oats

Bob's Red Mill Creamy Rice Hot Cereal, Millet Grits, Polenta (corn cereal) or "Mighty Tasty" Gluten-Free Hot Cereal (a combination of brown rice, corn, "sweet" white sorghum, and buckwheat) (all GF)

Lundberg Farms Hot 'n Creamy Rice Cereal (plain, unsweetened) (GF)

Pocono Cream of Buckwheat (GF)

Muesli

Earth Song Grandpa's Secret Omega-3 Muesli (made with quinoa flakes and chock-full of nuts, flaxseeds, dried fruits, and rice protein powder) (GF); another variety available with oats and quinoa flakes (not GF). (To prepare the muesli, soak it in water, gluten-free almond milk, or part water and light coconut milk or yogurt.)

Frozen Gluten-Free Waffles

Van's wheat-free, gluten-free waffles (available in original, blueberry, apple-cinnamon, and wheat-free with flax, the new, most nutritious variety) (GF)

Trader Joe's wheat-free, gluten-free waffles (GF)

Lifestream Mesa Sunrise or Buckwheat Wildberry waffles (GF, but both are made with corn)

Breads

French Meadow Bakery 100% rye sourdough bread with sunflower seeds or flaxseeds

Rudolph's 100% rye sourdough bread in several varieties

Food for Life Brown Rice Bread, Rice Almond Bread, Rice Pecan Bread, and Raisin Pecan Bread (best flavor when toasted) (GF)

Garden of Eatin' corn or blue corn mini-tortillas (GF, but made from corn)

Grain Side Dishes

Ancient Harvest or Arrowhead Mills Quinoa (GF)

Lundberg Farms Brown Rice, Country Wild, Wehani, Jubilee, and Wild Blends (blends of assorted whole-grain rices) (GF)

Lotus Foods Forbidden Rice and Bhutanese Red Rice (GF—and very colorful!)

Lowell Farms Organic Brown Jasmine Rice

Any brand of unseasoned brown basmati rice or wild rice (GF)

Pasta

Lundberg Organic Brown Rice Pasta, in linguini, penne, and other varieties (GF)

Tinkyada Brown Rice Pasta in a variety of shapes (GF)

Pastariso rice pasta in a variety of shapes (GF)

Ancient Harvest Quinoa Spaghetti with Corn, in a variety of shapes (GF, but contains corn)

Frozen Pizza

Nature's Hilights Organic Brown Rice Pizza Crust (you top it yourself; best to coat bottom of crust with a little olive oil to prevent sticking) (GF)

Nature's Hilights Italian Cheese, Soy Cheese, or Tostada Pizza: premade and ready to heat up (GF)

Cookies

Pamela's Products Gourmet Wheat-Free and Gluten-Free Cookies and Biscottis (the hands-down favorite in this department; they have dense textures and many tasty flavors, such as pecan shortbread, ginger cookies, peanut butter cookies, chocolate chip cookies, and almond anise biscotti) (all GF, except the oatmeal cookies)

Jennie's Coconut Macaroons (GF)

Baking Mixes and Supplies

Most gluten-free baking mixes are made with nutrient-poor ingredients, such as white rice flour, potato starch, tapioca starch, cornstarch, and sugar. I can't recommend them. Others contain corn, bean, and/or soy flours, which tend to cause digestive upset in many people.

Instead of working so hard to create breads, cookies, and other baked items that approximate wheat-based baked goods, it's better to wean yourself away from baked goods, eat more vegetables, and only occasionally make simple recipes for treats, special brunch foods, or holidays. The following are a few supplies that are needed to make some of the pancake and dessert recipes in Chapter 16.

Featherweight Cereal-Free, Gluten-Free Baking Powder (GF)

Arrowhead Mills or Bob's Red Mill Brown Rice, Millet, or Buckwheat Flours (GF)

Lotus Foods' Forbidden Rice, Bhutanese Red Rice, or Roasted Kaipen Rice Flour (GF)

Crackers

Kavli 100% rye, thin crispbread

Wasa Light Rye crispbread and Wasa Sourdough Rye crispbread

Any brand of wheat-free, gluten-free papadums (crispy, light Indian crackers made with bean flour and rice flour, or lentil flour) (GF)

Occasional Cheats from the Rules for Parties

Most crackers and chips are high in carbohydrates and undesirable fats—an unhealthy combination that packs on the pounds quickly. These products are best avoided except for an occasional splurge at a party. The following are some of the better choices in this category.

> Blue Diamond Nut Thins (an exception to the no-white-rice-flour rule because they contain nuts. Available in almond, hazelnut, and pecan varieties) (GF)
>
> Garden of Eatin' Blue Corn or Red Corn Chips (an improvement over traditional corn chips because they're organic) (GF, but contain corn)
>
> Olive Oil Potato Chips by Good Health Natural Foods (an improvement over regular potato chips because they're made with olive oil) (GF)
>
> Sweet Potato Chips and Exotic Vegetable Chips by Terra (a sneaky way of having kids and fussy adults eat more vegetables) (GF)

Shopping by Mail Order

If you don't have a health food store near you, you can order many products over the phone or Internet and have them shipped to you. I often recommend that my clients order unrefined oils and coconut butter directly from Omega Nutrition to get the freshest, highest quality oils possible.

For a complete listing of gluten-free baked goods and snacks that can be ordered, see www.GFMall.com. Special-ordering foods can be helpful if you have trouble finding certain products in your area, but remember that the products listed at this site should be ordered judiciously. You need to be just as savvy a shopper over the phone or Internet as you are in the grocery store.

CHAPTER 11

Eating Out
Against the Grain

E ating out against the grain can be difficult and discouraging, or it can be rewarding and fairly easy, depending on your specific dietary needs and attitude.
If you feel sorry for yourself and think of all the foods you're missing instead of all the delicious foods you can have, you probably won't enjoy
yourself much when you eat away from home. On the other hand, if you
let go of your former way of eating (which wasn't healthy to begin with)
and embrace eating out against the grain with gusto and resourcefulness,
this new way of eating becomes progressively easier and pays off in tasty
meals and health benefits you never imagined.

The good news is because of what you learned in the last chapter, you
already have gained much of the health-enhancing knowledge you need
to know to eat out against the grain. *The foods that are problems in grocery
stores are the same foods that can be problems in restaurants and at other
places away from home.* If you steer clear of those problem foods and look
and ask for creative combinations of nongrain foods, you'll be eating out
against the grain. This chapter will help you transfer your against-the-
grain know-how to different settings and fine-tune your skills so that you
can eat against the grain whenever you're away from home.

Eating Against the Grain in Restaurants

Restaurants were originally places where sickly customers were served highly concentrated broths made from meat and vegetables that had purported medicinal properties. Customers literally came to restaurants to be "restored."

Considering their origins, it is ironic that many restaurants today serve hidden and not-so-hidden sources of grains that can make people sick. If grain- and carbohydrate-sensitive people aren't careful about what they order in restaurants, they have to avoid restaurants and eat at home to have their health restored and maintained.

By ordering against the grain, you can make the restaurants that you visit approximate the spirit in which restaurants were originally created. When you ask the right questions and order mostly meat-and-vegetable combinations, restaurants can provide dining experiences that will support your physical health *and* your psychological health (by giving you a break from the regular cooking routine).

Against-the-Grain Restaurant Basics

Except for rye bread (which has wheat in it) and oatmeal, refined wheat is just about the only gluten grain ever found in choices in restaurants. That means that no matter whether you have wheat sensitivity, gluten sensitivity, or carbohydrate sensitivity, your strategy is pretty much the same: avoid wheat. To order against the grain, just get into the habit of saying no bun, no bread, no rolls, no tortillas, no croutons, no pasta, no flour, and no soy sauce, as circumstances warrant. Because of the recent popularity of low-carbohydrate diets, these types of requests are usually treated routinely.

The best entrée to order for any of the against-the-grain diets is fish, seafood, chicken, turkey, lean red meats, or game meat that is baked, broiled, steamed, stewed, sautéed, or poached—and at least two servings of vegetables. If you're carbohydrate sensitive, this is the easiest way to get a low-carbohydrate meal (providing you order nonstarchy vegetables). If you're wheat or gluten sensitive, this is the easiest way to get a safe meal without traces of gluten (providing the meat or fish isn't coated in flour, topped with a sauce made with flour, or marinated in something that contains gluten). If you aren't carbohydrate sensitive and want rice or potatoes with your meal, make sure they aren't prepared with flour or made in a broth or sauce that contains flour. Once you get these rules down, the rest is pretty much rudimentary.

Finding Good Restaurants, Calling Ahead, and Checking Out the Menu

There are lots of different restaurants out there, and some offer grain-based foods galore and not much else. To avoid arriving at a restaurant's doorstep for a meal and being disappointed by the choices it offers, check out the menu first.

There are several ways to do this. One is to call ahead and ask some questions at a time when the restaurant isn't busy—for example, 11 A.M. or 3 or 4 P.M. A far better way, especially if you are extremely sensitive to grains or have celiac disease, is to stop by the restaurant and pick up a menu. Or, if the restaurant has a Web page, go to the site and print out its menu. My favorite way is to call the restaurant and have someone fax a copy to me.

As you're looking over the menu, jot down questions that come to you, for example: Is this entrée made with flour? Can it be made without flour? What type of vegetable side dishes can I get instead of pasta? Then call the restaurant during off hours and talk to the chef, cook, or manager. This may seem like a big hassle, but it's becoming easier and easier. An increasing number of people in the restaurant business are becoming aware that many people can't tolerate gluten. Furthermore, most restaurant personnel (and chefs of good restaurants in particular) are sincere in wanting to make customers happy with tasty, satisfying meals. (They certainly don't want to cause customers to get sick!) As long as you are considerate by calling at a slow time and are polite about explaining what you need to avoid, chefs, cooks, and managers are often very willing to help.

Talking to the chef or manager beforehand is particularly important when you're dining out for special occasions, such as birthdays and anniversaries. If you give chefs of good restaurants enough notice, you can often make special arrangements for gluten-free cakes and desserts or low-carbohydrate desserts. (Sure, these desserts have white sugar, but eating a bit of sugar on very special occasions is no big deal, especially compared to how much worse it would be to eat refined sugar and refined wheat together!) Being able to indulge in specially prepared desserts can be a godsend for helping you (or your loved ones) enjoy festive occasions in good physical and emotional health.

One last point to keep in mind: If you talk with several people at a restaurant and each one is uncooperative, unhelpful, and maybe downright rude, explain your disappointment at not being able to try their restaurant and take your business elsewhere. This doesn't happen often, but you should be prepared if it does. You're the customer; restaurants should be in the business of making customers happy. If people at a restaurant don't have this philosophy, it isn't a place you want to patronize. Try to reward restaurants that treat you well by visiting them frequently, getting to know the personnel by name, and thanking them (with words and nice tips) for great meals and great service.

General Guidelines for Ordering in Different Kinds of Restaurants

Whether you call ahead or just stop in spontaneously, certain foods are no-nos in every restaurant and certain foods you can be fairly sure are free of grains. (I say "fairly sure" because chefs often put their own unique stamps on standard recipes. When in doubt, ask.) The tips that follow take you through the basics of healthy foods to order and grain-laced foods to avoid in a variety of different restaurants.

A special caveat, though: The suggestions should be helpful for most people who are wheat sensitive, gluten sensitive, or carbohydrate sensitive. However, they do not cover every conceivable way trace amounts of gluten or grain-based additives can slip into your food. (One example: cooking gluten-free food on a grill or frying it in a fryer where other gluten foods have been cooked can leave trace amounts that some people may react to.) So, *use these recommendations at your discretion.* If you are a celiac or grain-allergic person who is extremely sensitive to trace amounts of grains, I strongly suggest that you work with a celiac or food allergy support group or a grain-savvy nutritionist and learn how to be extra diligent about protecting your health.

In American-Style and Hotel Restaurants

Breakfast

Eggs and fruit are by far the best against-the-grain choices on the menu. You can get eggs prepared virtually any way, and you usually can get beneficial vegetables as well: look for omelets that contain vegetables or combinations of scrambled eggs and vegetables—for example, spinach and onion omelets, or huevos rancheros (Mexican-style eggs with peppers, onions, chiles, tomatoes, and often a little cheese). If you don't see anything like this, ask your server. Hotel restaurants in particular almost always have vegetables on hand, so the staff can usually make egg-and-vegetable combinations without much trouble. Hollandaise sauce, made from egg yolks, butter, and lemon juice, can be a nice, gluten-free egg topper for extra flavor.

Hash brown potatoes can also be ordered if you're not carbohydrate sensitive. Try poached eggs on hash brown potatoes instead of bread. Oatmeal, a wheat-free food but not a gluten-free food, is another option.

Obtaining concentrated protein in the morning is critical for stabilizing blood sugar. Unfortunately, there aren't as many options in this area

---

An Against-the-Grain Breakfast

If you are carbohydrate sensitive:
Spinach and onion omelet with hollandaise sauce
Side dish of strawberries

If you aren't carbohydrate sensitive:
2 poached eggs on hashed brown potatoes
$1/2$ grapefruit

as there should be. Breakfast steaks are sometimes available, or try making a special request for a broiled chicken breast. This may seem like a strange order for breakfast, but it really is a great way to start the day, and it's often a request that's fairly easy for hotel restaurants to accommodate.

If you're carbohydrate sensitive, other protein foods, such as low-fat cottage cheese, ham, Canadian bacon, and lox or smoked salmon, can work well in a pinch. Keep in mind that some of these foods contain additives or ingredients that may bother some people. To help protect against the harmful effects of some of the additives these foods contain, eat breakfast meats with vitamin C–rich fruits, or take vitamin C and vitamin E supplements with them.

Lunch

Soup, sandwiches, and salad are standard fare on many lunch menus. Soup should always be on the automatic "no" list unless you can verify that the soup is homemade without any flour, commercial stocks, or bouillons used as starters.

Burgers, turkey burgers, and grilled chicken sandwiches can easily turn into against-the-grain choices: just remember to say "no bun" or "no bread." In fancier places, "no focaccia" (an upscale kind of bread) may be in order. As a side dish with the meat or chicken, order a salad, steamed vegetables, or fruit salad—or a baked potato (if you can afford the extra carbohydrate calories) or cole slaw (if you do okay with vinegar).

Salads are great ways to get a lot of vegetables and eat against the grain. The main things you have to watch out for are croutons; tortillas (which sometimes come sliced on Mexican-style salads); oriental or Chinese salads, which are made with soy sauce and often contain wheat-

---

An Against-the-Grain Lunch

Grilled chicken and portabello mushroom sandwich
    with no bread or focaccia
Steamed broccoli
Side of sliced fresh melon or fruit salad

based noodles; breaded chicken, which occasionally arrives on top of salads instead of grilled chicken; marinated chicken; blue cheese and roquefort cheese, which are often made with wheat; and processed cheese or processed sour cream, which sometimes contains gluten additives. Despite these restrictions, there should be plenty of choices; for example, grilled shrimp salad, chicken cobb salad, or spinach salad without the blue cheese and bacon bits.

If white vinegar doesn't bother you, all salad dressings except blue cheese, roquefort, soy-sauce-based dressings (such as peanut dressings), and sweet dressings (such as sweet and sour) may be acceptable choices in moderation. (Mustard-based dressings may be bothersome to some.) However, commercial salad dressings tend to have unhealthy oils and additives, so it's best to order them on the side and use them sparingly, or thin them out with lemon juice or olive oil. The safest choices are always olive oil and red wine vinegar, balsamic vinegar, or lemon wedges, followed by red wine, balsamic, or citrus vinaigrettes.

Dinner

If you find yourself hungry while waiting for meals and watching others eat bread, carry a bag of nuts in your purse or briefcase with you and snack on them while you're waiting for your entrée to arrive. Don't let complimentary bread tempt you. Always tell the waiter or the busboy not to bring it to your table, and take comfort in the fact that it's going on someone else's waistline, not yours. If the dipping sauce is really tempting (for example, basil- and garlic-infused olive oil), ask your waiter if you could have a side dish of veggie sticks.

An Against-the-Grain Dinner

Dinner salad with tomatoes, cucumber, shredded carrot, red cabbage, and olive oil and red wine vinegar
Roasted chicken with rosemary
Zucchini, yellow squash, and carrot medley

It usually is easy in a hotel or American–style restaurant to get some type of baked or broiled meat, poultry, or fish entrée with vegetables and a nice, fresh salad. Roasted chicken, steaks, grilled (unbreaded) pork chops, grilled shrimp, and baked or broiled fish are all good choices. Be sure to avoid items listed with the wheat-based culinary terms on page 193 and avoid sweet dishes made with sugar. If you don't know how certain foods are prepared, be sure to ask for more specifics.

Dessert

Refined wheat goes hand in hand with refined sugar in almost all desserts. That means there are two good health reasons to avoid dessert on a regular basis.

If you feel the need for a bite of dessert on special occasions, seek out gluten-free desserts. Fruit sorbet, some types of ice cream, berries, and real whipped cream, crème brûlée, chocolate mousse, and flourless chocolate cake usually all qualify—however, make sure the cake pan is not dusted with flour. If you're not especially gluten sensitive, you might also be able to eat the filling of fruit pies and pumpkin pie (and avoid the crust) without running into trouble. Keep in mind, though, that many of these desserts contain milk products, which can cause as many health problems as grains for some people.

The best dessert, of course, is fruit. Packed with nutrients and refreshing, fruit doesn't cause a bloated and overstuffed feeling like typical desserts do. A dish of mixed berries is an especially good choice. Even if fruit isn't on the menu, ask for it: many restaurants can put a dish together.

Seafood Restaurants

In seafood restaurants, you can order many different types of healthful fish, including varieties you hardly ever have the opportunity to eat. Fish that are particularly rich in beneficial omega-3 fatty acids are anchovies, Atlantic cod, Atlantic salmon, haddock, halibut, king salmon, mackerel, rainbow trout, and tuna.

When ordering, watch out for breaded, crusted, or encrusted fish, fish with cream sauces, and fish prepared with soy sauce. Pan-fried dishes, such as sole amandine or trout amandine are usually coated in

Wheat by Any Other Name

Besides obvious items that contain wheat (bread, breaded items, buns, bagels, croutons, and flour tortillas), there are lots of other places wheat can hide on a restaurant menu. The following are some of the most common culinary terms for food items and methods of preparation that involve wheat.

Au gratin (made with bread crumbs and cheese)

Batter-dipped foods, such as fish

Beef Wellington

Beignet (a dessert fritter popular in Louisiana)

Bisque (a thick soup)

Couscous (a wheat-based side dish in Middle Eastern and African cuisine)

Cream sauces, cream soups, gravies, and roux-based dishes

Crepe (a thin, wheat-based pancake used in desserts and entrées)

Focaccia (a fancy Italian bread with herbs)

Fried (as in fried zucchini, fried chicken, and pan-fried fish)

Gnocchi (Italian potato dumplings that contain wheat)

Heavy dishes, including à la king (as in chicken à la king), casseroles, goulash, fricassee (as in chicken fricassee), Kiev (as in chicken Kiev), Newburg (as in lobster Newburg), and stroganoff (as in beef stroganoff)

Loaf (as in meatloaf or turkey loaf), meatballs (typically made with bread crumbs), and patties (as in fish patties)

Polonnaise (a method of food preparation involving bread crumbs)

Quiche

Stuffed entrées and side dishes (as in stuffed flounder or mushrooms)

Tempura

An Against-the-Grain Seafood Dinner

Green leafy salad topped with baby shrimp and red wine vinaigrette

Rainbow trout amandine prepared without flour

Green beans

flour before they're cooked, but they can almost always be prepared without it if you ask. Some of the best choices to order are fish prepared with olive oil, lemon, and herbs or with various butters, such as dill butter, garlic butter, lemon butter, or caper butter. Other gluten-free sauces for fish are fruit salsa, salsa, and pesto sauce.

Italian Restaurants

The trick to avoiding pizza, bread, and pasta in Italian restaurants is to go to a nice Italian restaurant that offers meatier entrées and tasty salads and vegetable side dishes. Many chicken and veal dishes (such as chicken picatta and veal scallopini) may be made with flour, but chefs can make these dishes without flour if you request it.

Although styles vary from restaurant to restaurant, Italian entrées that are usually gluten free include chicken aioli (in olive oil, black olives, Italian herbs, garlic, and white wine); chicken lemone (in lemon garlic butter); pollo arrosto (roast chicken with rosemary or other herbs); chicken cacciatore (in a marinara sauce with peppers and onions); shrimp scampi in garlic butter, olive oil, or marinara sauce; minestrone or cioppino made without pasta; and sometimes scallops, mussels, veal chops, or lamb chops. Some Italian restaurants also offer whole fresh fish or fish filets oven baked with flavorful vegetables, olives, olive oil, and herbs with or without tomato sauce. This is a real treat when you can find it.

For side dishes, look for roasted asparagus with balsamic vinegar, sautéed spinach, steamed artichoke with a vinaigrette dressing, a medley of flavorful grilled or sautéed vegetables, or any one of a number of tasty salads. If you can afford the extra carbohydrates in your diet, other wheat-

---

An Against-the-Grain Italian Dinner

Shrimp scampi lemone (in lemon and garlic butter) or shrimp
scampi provencale (with black olives, artichokes, mushrooms,
tomato, garlic, and herbs)
Roasted asparagus with balsamic vinegar
Sautéed spinach with garlic

---

free options are risotto (from rice) and polenta (from corn). One dessert
that tends to be gluten free is zabaglione, a whipped concoction made
from egg yolks.

Greek Restaurants

Greek restaurants are one of the easiest places to eat against the grain.
Sure, there are some grainy trouble spots: pita bread; spanakopita
(spinach pie); tyropita (cheese pie); pasta dishes, such as orzo and pastit-
sio (macaroni dish); moussaka (an eggplant-meat dish made with
béchamel sauce); saganaki (flamed cheese made with bread crumbs);
gyros (a garlicky lamb-beef mixture where wheat is often hidden); and
Greek pastries. But bypass those, and you won't believe the delicious food
you can have.

First, there are the appetizers: hummus (a garlicky sesame–chick pea
dip); tzatziki (yogurt dip with cucumbers, lemon juice, garlic, and
onion); and baba ghanoush (roasted eggplant dip with garlic and lemon).
To enjoy them, ask for a side order of sliced cucumbers, which is always
available in Greek kitchens (or if you prefer, bring your own gluten-free
crackers). Greek salad or village salad (without lettuce) are almost always
dressed in olive oil and red wine vinegar or lemon juice, so they're naturally gluten free.

When it comes to Greek entrées, there are choices galore, including
broiled lamb chops with garlic and herbs; roast leg of lamb; lamb shanks
(they shouldn't be dredged in flour, but ask); chicken Athenian (Hellenic
lemon chicken); broiled Greek-style fish (with olive oil, herbs, and

An Against-the-Grain Greek Dinner

Appetizer of cucumber slices with baba ghanoush

Roast leg of lamb or lamb shank with lemon, garlic, and herbs

Sautéed asparagus in olive oil with herbs

Sautéed greens in olive oil with garlic

garlic); scallops or shrimp scampi in olive oil and garlic; and lamb, pork, beef, chicken, and seafood souvlaki (kabobs drizzled with olive oil and herbs and often skewered with tasty vegetables). Dolmas—grape leaves stuffed with rice and ground beef—should be gluten free. Order them without the avgolemono sauce if the sauce is made with wheat.

Side dishes often include sautéed asparagus, zucchini, and peppers; sautéed greens in olive oil with herbs; and green beans in tomato sauce. Higher carbohydrate choices are Greek potato salad, roasted potatoes with olive oil and lemon, and skorthalia (whipped potatoes with olive oil and garlic). These side dishes are so dreamy, you can treat them like dessert! If you really want a bite of dessert, two wheat-free choices are rice pudding and halvah, a ground sesame-honey candy.

Middle Eastern Restaurants

Middle Eastern restaurants, such as Lebanese, Jordanian, Armenian, and Turkish eateries, use slightly different spices than those used in Greek cuisines, but they offer similar gluten-free choices on the menu. Among the choices are hummus, eggplant dip, stuffed grape leaves, stuffed cabbage, chicken and lamb dishes, and lots of different types of kabobs. Schwarma, another offering, is often made with chicken, beef, or lamb kabob meat and topped with hummus or tahini sauce, sliced onions, and tomato. It usually is served in pita bread, but it's easy for the cook not to use the pita. Be careful to avoid couscous and tabouli, both made from wheat, as well as falafels (fried, breaded, ground chickpea mixtures).

An Against-the-Grain Middle Eastern Dinner

Appetizer of stuffed grape leaves

Chicken kabob or chicken schwarma with no pita

Salad with lettuce, cucumber, olive oil, lemon juice, and herbs

Moroccan restaurants differ a bit. They often offer dishes made with honey and dried fruits. While gluten free, these dishes are often overly sweet—more like dessert than a blood-sugar-stabilizing meal—so it's best to avoid them. Kabobs are usually the healthiest choices on the menu, followed by nonsweet tagines (mixtures of vegetables, olive oil, and assorted spices, or preserved lemon and olive oil).

French or Other Continental Restaurants

The bad news about French and Continental cuisine is that most dishes are made with flour. The good news is that many of them, such as sautéed chicken breasts, veal medallions, or many fish dishes (often in wine sauces), can be made without wheat if you specifically request it. Tell your server right off the bat that you can't have wheat. Ask him to check with the chef about which items don't have wheat and which ones can be made without it. Another good strategy is to look for something simple on the menu.

A number of salads, such as wilted spinach salad, caesar salad without the croutons, and salade nicoise (made with tuna, new potatoes, green beans, olives, tomatoes, and vinaigrette dressing) shouldn't contain wheat. Other items that either are wheat free or can be made that way include poached salmon, fish en papillote (fish cooked in its own juices with herbs); bouillabaisse (seafood stew); sea scallops in garlic butter; mussels cooked in white wine, garlic, and herbs; mixed grill (a trio of grilled meats and/or seafood); poulet aux fines herbes (roast chicken with herbs); ratatouille (eggplant-tomato side dish); roasted new potatoes; and duck à l'orange (a sweet dish that's good on occasion for a treat, but not recommended if you are carbohydrate sensitive).

An Against-the-Grain
French or Continental Dinner

Wilted spinach salad with mushrooms, artichoke hearts, and
red wine vinaigrette dressing

Bouillabaisse (clear-broth fish and shellfish stew with white
wine, tomatoes, onions, garlic, and herbs, verified to be
free of flour or commercial stock) *or*

Mixed grill with no sauces and roasted asparagus

Mexican Restaurants

If you're in the mood for Mexican food, it pays to go to a nice Mexican restaurant. Cheap places offer grain-heavy meals without a lot of meat but with a lot of salt, additives, and unhealthy processed cheese (which often contains gluten).

In a nice Mexican restaurant, you can find simply prepared dishes, such as camarones al mojo de ajo (shrimp sautéed in olive oil and garlic); red snapper or sea bass prepared Veracruz style (with tomatoes, onions, and peppers); grilled fish tacos with salsa and guacamole (with no tortillas); grilled fish with fruit salsa or bean-based sauces; pork loin in roasted tomatillo sauce; and chicken in mole sauces (which usually do not contain gluten). Carne asada and chicken, fish, or beef fajitas (without the tortillas) are other good choices, providing there isn't anything problematic in the seasoning.

Salads with dressings such as cilantro-lime vinaigrettes can usually be found, along with sautéed or grilled zucchini and peppers, or jicama

An Against-the-Grain Mexican Dinner

Grilled fish taco with salsa and guacamole and no tortillas

Grilled zucchini and peppers

Jicama salad

salad side dishes. Beans, rice, and corn tortillas are also available if you tolerate them.

Oriental Restaurants

In Oriental restaurants, including Japanese, Chinese, and Thai, MSG and soy sauces hide in many types of foods, so it's important to be extremely careful when looking over the menu and ordering. Some sensitive types do best avoiding these restaurants altogether.

In Japanese restaurants, soy-sauce-based ingredients are everywhere—from teriyaki and sukiyaki preparations to tofu dishes and sometimes miso. Your safest bet for avoiding gluten is to choose sashimi or sushi (seafood or seafood-and-rice combinations rolled in seaweed). Unfortunately, there's one big drawback and danger to these dishes: Most of the fish is served raw, so there's a risk of parasitic contamination that can cause severe illness. To eliminate this risk, I strongly urge you to opt for sushi made from cooked shrimp, crab, eel, octopus, or egg. This is especially important if you suffer from digestive trouble, as many celiacs and gluten-sensitive people do. To avoid the soy sauce that comes with the sushi, bring wheat-free tamari from home or try a tiny bit of wasabi (made with vinegar and horseradish).

In Chinese restaurants, steer clear of deep-fried and breaded entrées; pickled items; fried rice (made with soy sauce); and soy, hoisin, plum, and sweet-and-sour sauces (which contain wheat and sugar). What's left? Stir-fries with chicken and vegetables in clear sauces thickened with cornstarch (if you aren't sensitive)—that means dishes such as moo goo gai pan—or dishes that the chef prepares especially for you.

Often the easiest way around the hidden ingredients in Oriental cooking is to go to a Mongolian stir-fry place and select your own meat and vegetable ingredients. The employees will cook your dish right in front of you on a hot rock or grill in just a few minutes. The downside of Mongolian barbecues is that traces of soy sauce from previous dishes may end up in other dishes. So, if you have celiac disease or are extremely allergic, eating at Mongolian stir-fry places isn't for you. However, if you are carbohydrate sensitive or only mildly wheat sensitive, Mongolian barbecues can

---

An Against-the-Grain Oriental Meal

Moo goo gai pan (chicken sautéed with pea pods,
bamboo shoots, mushrooms, and carrots) *or*
Mongolian-grilled stir-fry with meats and vegetables of
your choosing

---

often be healthy choices, especially when you want something fast that is
rich in vegetables. To give your stir-fries nice flavor without soy sauce,
load your dish up with onions, peppers, garlic water, ginger water,
cilantro, and—if you like—cashews and sesame oil. Bring a small shaker
of unrefined salt with you from home to salt your dish and avoid the hazards of commercial table salt.

Eating Against the Grain on the Run

In the fast-paced world we live in, many of us have gotten into the habit
of plopping wheat-based convenience foods into our mouths when we're
hungry. Quick as this way of eating is, it's a big reason for the widespread
development of carbohydrate sensitivity, gluten sensitivity, and wheat
sensitivity.

To eat against the grain and revitalize our health, we have to break
ourselves of this habit, find better alternatives for fast food on the run,
and take a bit more time to plan ahead.

The Hazards of Typical Fast Food

Fast-food restaurants offer food that is a major source of hidden sugar,
salt, additives, and nonessential fat. For that reason alone, you should
avoid eating at these places. But there's another reason: many foods—
even simple things like grilled chicken from inside a chicken sandwich—
have hidden forms of wheat and gluten. In addition, some fast-food
companies will do anything to keep from disclosing their ingredients. So,

caveat emptor (let the buyer beware). If you have celiac disease or a strong grain allergy, you can't afford to play Russian roulette with your health. The safest thing is always to plan ahead so you won't be forced to visit these restaurants when you're starved.

If you're carbohydrate sensitive but not particularly gluten sensitive, you can get away with more, such as ordering a big burger with lettuce, tomato and mustard and no bun and a salad at a burger place. Or you can order a salad, steamed vegetables, and rotisserie chicken (remove the skin before eating) at a chicken place. But if you have to take a chance on choosing food that may have a touch of wheat, I think it's better to go to the Mongolian barbecue and have a stir fry your way, loaded up with healthful vegetables.

Healthier Fast Food

Far better choices are to pick up convenient meat-and-vegetable combinations at health food stores. At most of the major natural food supermarkets, there are salad bars and big deli cases featuring simply prepared rotisserie chicken; roast pork or beef; grilled salmon; grilled or steamed vegetables; gluten-free, antibiotic-free deli meats from Applegate Farms and other brands; and a wide variety of chicken, turkey, potato, and vegetable salads—many of which are gluten free. Most ingredients are clearly listed, and employees are quite helpful answering questions about how foods are prepared. Order carefully, and you can pick up fast food with confidence.

Buying ready-to-eat items from the natural foods supermarket is a great way to get a quick meal on the go. If you buy some deli items ahead of time and put them in your refrigerator, you can also have food around your house that can turn into a fast meal later in the week.

Homemade Fast Food

If you don't have a natural foods supermarket near your home or work, or if you need to avoid a lot of ingredients, another option is to make your own fast food. Try to make this as easy as possible by making extra of foods you're preparing for dinners. For example, save leftover meat from

a roasted turkey to top lettuce salads or to make turkey salad or sandwiches. Make a big pot of soup or a big stir-fry and heat up the leftovers
later in the week. Or broil a bunch of turkey or chicken kabobs for dinner, then cut up the leftover meat and vegetables (usually red onion, peppers, and mushrooms), put them in a bowl, and pour vinaigrette dressing
over the mixture. There's your ready-to-eat turkey or chicken salad for to-
morrow. To take cold or hot foods with you wherever you may need
them—at work, on picnics, on day trips, or while racing around town
shopping and doing chores—invest in an insulated lunch cold pack and
a thermos.

Portable Snacks

Always get into the habit of carrying snacks with you. Even if you think
you're going to be away from home for only an hour or two, unexpected
things can happen and schedules can change. For example, your car
could break down or you could find an incredible sale on clothing that
you just can't pass up. Either way, you can't afford to get in a jam and eat
the only food you can find, which undoubtedly would be a wheat-based
food. So, prepare for those times when life is unpredictable: regularly
carry snack foods with you.

Nuts and seeds are the best snack foods I know. They are portable,
convenient, sturdy, and ready to eat; free of wheat, gluten, and other
problematic grains; rich in healthy fat, carbohydrates, protein, vitamins,
and minerals; and stabilizing to blood sugar (and energy) levels. Plus,
they come in lots of different varieties. Macadamia nuts are particularly
good for stabilizing blood sugar, but any kind of nut will do. An apple—
a hardy, filling fruit—often makes a nice companion to nuts.

Other good snack foods are often nut related, such as trail mixes, Nu-
tiva nut bars (found in health food stores), nut butter sandwiches on
gluten-free bread or crackers, celery sticks spread with nut butter, and
Amaretto Protein Bars (see recipe in Chapter 15). However, the first three
are higher in carbohydrates and aren't appropriate for people who are carbohydrate sensitive. (They are better than candy bars or cookies, though!)
The latter two aren't quite as convenient or sturdy as nuts. Unfortunately,

there isn't a commercial protein bar I can recommend; most contain grain or have too much sugar. If you find a sugar- and grain-free protein bar that you like and do well with, go ahead and use it as an occasional snack food.

Eating Against the Grain on the Road

When you're traveling, all the creature comforts of home aren't with you. Plus, you can encounter lots of unexpected curves on the road and in the "friendly" skies. That means it's more important than ever to plan ahead and take handy foods with you.

Some people may bring a few foods (such as nuts), then wing it the rest of the way, relying on their skills for ordering against the grain in restaurants. Others may need or choose to go further by packing a small compactible, soft-sided cooler or surfing the Internet to learn about the best restaurant choices in the area they will be visiting. (I always look for Greek restaurants!) Still others, such as some celiacs, plan complete gluten-free cruises and travel getaways to ensure no gluten slip-ups on their vacations. How far you go to eat against the grain on the road should be a matter of your individual preference and needs. The suggestions that follow are some simple general guidelines.

Traveling by Car

When you take a road trip, you have the luxury of packing a big cooler with deli meats, gluten-free sandwiches, deli salads, veggie sticks, fruit, and lots of water. This will give you a few ready-to-eat meals on the road, so you won't have to stop at a hazardous-to-your-health fast-food joint. If you have a way to refreeze your blue ice on your trip, you can buy more food during your trip. This is especially important if you are planning a day in the great outdoors.

Traveling by Plane

To make it easier to eat against the grain while flying, call your airline several days before your flight and order something special. Special meals are not perfect, but they certainly are a great improvement over standard meals, which are loaded with refined wheat, salt, sugar, unhealthy fat, and additives. The following is a description of the best against-the-grain choices in special meals.

Gluten Free

Gluten-free special meals are the way to go if you need to strictly avoid wheat or all gluten. Gluten-free meals are offered on virtually all North American airlines, except Alaska Airlines, America West, and Southwest.

Gluten-free lunches and dinners differ from airline to airline, but they usually include chicken, shrimp, fish, or beef; a salad with gluten-free dressing; rice or potatoes; and sometimes fruit. In place of the roll and dessert on standard meals, airlines typically include a couple of fat-free rice cakes and some type of gluten-free sugary concoction. Avoid these products: they can send your blood sugar soaring through very unhappy skies. Stick with the protein and vegetables and round out this meal with nuts brought from home.

Cold gluten-free breakfasts often entail a corn-based cereal or corn muffin, a rice cake, and fruit—in other words, a high-carbohydrate, blood-sugar-raising meal, which is a disastrous way to start a trip. Hot breakfasts are a little better: they usually include fruit, potatoes, and an omelette (although, I'm sorry to say, on some major airlines the omelette is made from fake eggs, not real eggs). My advice would be to eat something rich in protein at home before you head to the airport, skip the cold breakfast in favor of the fruit plate, and supplement the hot breakfast offerings with nuts or other good snack foods.

Fruit Plate

Fresh fruit plates are offered for all meals on all flights. The fruit is really quite good—it is refreshing and gives you lots of protective nutrients. Unfortunately, it doesn't give you staying power. To prevent low energy levels a few hours after eating, share your fruit plate with a traveling companion and balance the fruit with snack foods rich in protein and healthy fat.

Other Special Meals

Other options are available if you want to get a good meal but don't need to avoid every speck of wheat. To decide on the best choice for you, call an airline agent several days before your flight and ask if he or she could give you an idea of the kind of meal that might be served for the following choices: a gluten-free meal, a seafood plate, a diabetic meal, or a chef salad (on United Airlines only). The seafood plate is often the best choice (even when offered for breakfast, which is usually a seafood omelette), but all the choices can be good at times for eating against the grain. However, pasta, bread, and wheat-containing sauces and desserts can show up on most of these meals, so be prepared for this. Have the discipline to push aside any refined-wheat products on your plate.

Making Arrangements for Special Meals

You actually can order special meals at the same time you make your reservation with an airline. If you forget, call the airline a week ahead of time to request them. For extra insurance, call two days before your flight to confirm that your meals are on order.

Even when you do everything right, airlines sometimes can mess up special meal orders. If this happens, ask the flight attendant if there are any other special meals on board and not claimed: sometimes you can get lucky. If not, live off the snacks that you have brought until you find more suitable food. When things go awry on trips, nuts become lifesavers for staying away from grains.

Another Trick of Traveling

Try to stay in a hotel room that has a small refrigerator, if possible. When you call to make hotel reservations, ask if the rooms have refrigerators or mini-bars. If they don't, see if you can request one for no extra charge. Hotels often have a few on hand.

Having access to a refrigerator makes the room feel more homey. You can put leftovers from dinner in the refrigerator and have healthy fast food when you need it. I find this a survival skill that's especially important on long trips. There are limited gluten-free items on breakfast menus—and it gets boring to have eggs day after day after day—so I often have leftover chicken or meat pieces in place of eggs for variety.

If I know I'm going to have a refrigerator on a long trip, I bring along Earth Song gluten-free muesli, a can of coconut milk, a can opener, a spoon, and a small plastic bowl. Earth Song muesli is a great traveling food: it can be soaked at room temperature in water. However, I prefer to soak it in part water and coconut milk overnight in the refrigerator (and order up fresh pineapple from room service!). The muesli is enriched with rice protein powder and is chock-full of nuts and dried fruits, so it's a nice, light breakfast alternative.

You've learned all about how to shop against the grain in supermarkets and eat against the grain in restaurants, on the run, and on the road. Now it's time to get an idea of what a week's worth of meals in each of the against-the-grain diets should look like.

CHAPTER 12

The Totally Against-the-Grain Diet and Menu Plan

Now that you've prepared yourself both psychologically and practically to go against the grain, it's time to learn about the various against-the-grain diets. The Totally Against-the-Grain Diet will be covered first, even though it's the strictest diet. That's because more and more North Americans are developing serious problems with carbohydrate sensitivity that require strong dietary intervention, at least initially. The other two diets, discussed in the next two chapters, include some grains, starchy vegetables, and legumes and are a little higher in carbohydrates.

The Totally Against-the-Grain Diet is right for you if:

- You scored high on the Carbohydrate Sensitivity questionnaire.

- You have weight that hasn't budged on less strict eating plans.

- You have at least two indicators of Syndrome X (abdominal obesity, hypertension, high cholesterol, elevated triglycerides).

- You have polycystic ovary syndrome (PCOS).

- You have Type 2 diabetes.

Characteristics of the
Totally Against-the-Grain Diet

- Low carbohydrate

- Free of all grains, refined sugars, legumes, and starchy vegetables

- Rich in protein and monounsaturated and omega-3 fats

- You have tried either of the other two against-the-grain diet plans and have been unable to get the weight-loss results or improvements in blood pressure, cholesterol, triglycerides, or PCOS symptoms and indicators that you want.

The Totally Against-the-Grain Diet is low in carbohydrates and free of all grains and refined sugars. The carbohydrates come from low-glycemic, nonstarchy vegetables and small amounts of low-glycemic fruits and nuts. The diet is also rich in protein and heart-healthy monounsaturated and omega-3 fats. By replacing grains and other starchy foods with nonstarchy vegetables and quality fats, this diet stimulates better blood sugar and insulin metabolism at the same time it promotes satiety.

This diet is especially appropriate for people who have the conditions that were listed, but it's safe for almost anyone. Three big cautions, though: pregnant women, Type 1 diabetics, and those with impaired kidney function should not follow this diet without doctor supervision.

Although people who follow the Totally Against-the-Grain Diet should try to avoid all grain products (including grain-derived food additives), their primary focus should be to address carbohydrate sensitivity and keep carbohydrates low in the diet.

If a small amount of a grain-based ingredient or additive sneaks into a meal from time to time, this probably won't be a problem. However, if you're gluten sensitive, wheat sensitive, or corn sensitive, in addition to being carbohydrate sensitive, then you'll have to be more careful about watching out for and avoiding trace amounts of grains and grain additives.

Some people may do fine including low-carbohydrate milk products, such as cheese and whey protein powders, in this diet. However, animal studies suggest that milk protein may contribute to insulin resistance. To be on the safe side (and to show you how tasty foods can be without dairy), I did not include dairy foods in this sample menu plan. I suggest you try this diet without dairy for two weeks, evaluate how you feel, then add some butter and small amounts of cheese and see how you do. If you start to feel worse or gain weight by eating dairy products, realize that your body is telling you that dairy is not good for you, at least not right now. Heed these signs.

Lastly, keep in mind that this is a *sample* menu. It does not have to be followed to the letter. Rather, it should be changed according to your needs. If you do not like a meat or nonstarchy vegetable that's listed in the menu, replace it with something similar. Just make sure to follow the against-the-grain diet guidelines, and keep your carbohydrate intake low. An asterisk (*) indicates that the recipe is included in Chapter 15.

THE TOTALLY AGAINST-THE-GRAIN DIET PLAN
One-Week Sample Menu

DAY 1

Breakfast	2 eggs scrambled with chopped mushrooms, sliced green onions, garlic, and dried basil sautéed in olive oil
Lunch	Small piece of broiled trout topped with toasted sliced almonds Sautéed green bok choy tops with garlic in olive oil
Dinner	Chicken Legs and Thighs Herbes de Provence* (one leg and one thigh) Roasted Asparagus* Romaine salad with chopped radish and cucumber topped with herbs, red wine vinegar, and olive oil

Snack (optional)   A handful of almonds

DAY 2

Breakfast   2 reheated Chicken Legs Herbes de Provence
Celery sticks with cashew butter

Lunch   Broiled turkey, buffalo, or organic beef burger
topped with sliced tomato and a dab of
guacamole
Cole slaw *or* Arizona Cole Slaw*

Dinner   Filet of Sole Florentine* with spinach, onions,
and lemon juice

Snack (optional)   Several Kalamata olives

DAY 3

Breakfast   Breakfast steak tidbits sautéed in olive oil with
onions, red peppers or julienne green beans,
garlic powder, and oregano

Lunch   Baked halibut with olive oil, dill, salt, and
pepper
Large spinach salad with a few toasted
hazelnuts or pecans and a few sliced
strawberries, topped with unrefined
hazelnut oil and balsamic vinegar

Dinner   Roast turkey breast slices with sage and
natural au jus
Steamed Brussels sprouts with lemon juice and
olive oil

Snack (optional)   A handful of macadamia nuts

DAY 4

Breakfast	Unsweetened, gluten-free chicken sausage ½ cup of blueberries
Lunch	Open-faced turkey sandwich (from leftover turkey) on a slice of Nut Protein Bread* with baby romaine lettuce leaves, a slice of avocado, and a dab of pesto sauce or mayonnaise
Dinner	Broiled lamb chops with garlic powder, oregano, salt, and pepper, sprinkled with lemon juice Sautéed mushrooms and zucchini with oregano and garlic in olive oil
Snack (optional)	Several green olives stuffed with garlic

DAY 5

Breakfast	2 eggs scrambled with chopped green pepper in olive oil
Lunch	Guacamole Shrimp Salad* with red pepper, shallot, and cilantro on a few romaine lettuce leaves
Dinner	Baked Pork Chops with Caraway Seeds and Cabbage*
Snack (optional)	A few jicama sticks with guacamole Leftover slice of meat of any type

DAY 6

Breakfast	Joe's Special* (scrambled eggs, hamburger meat, and spinach)
Lunch	Swordfish or chicken kabob with herbs Large romaine salad with 2 tomato wedges,

sliced cucumber, 4 diced olives, and 1 red onion slice, tossed with Fresh Basil Lemon-ette Dressing*

Dinner   Baked or broiled salmon with garlic powder, oregano, paprika, and a drizzle of olive oil and a wedge of lemon
Sautéed asparagus in olive oil with dill
Small cucumber and red onion salad with dill and sugar-free red wine vinaigrette

Snack (optional)   A handful of pumpkin seeds and a few berries *or* celery sticks with nut butter

DAY 7

Breakfast   Caraway Turkey Sausage Patties*
1 slice of Nut Protein Bread*

Lunch   Grecian Lamb Balls*
Steamed broccoli and cauliflower

Dinner   Shrimp or scallops sautéed in olive oil with garlic, spinach, sliced hearts of palm, dried oregano and basil, sprinkled with lemon juice

Snack (optional)   1 hard-boiled egg
A few radishes and cucumber slices

Sugar-Free Beverage Choices (from best to worst)

Filtered or bottled water, plain or with a lemon or lime wedge

Sparkling mineral water

Unsweetened, gluten-free herbal teas

Plain, unsweetened, unflavored green tea, red bush tea, or black tea

Plain coffee without sugar (no more than two cups per day)

Seeing Results

Most people start to see some improvements in health—say, a loss of a few pounds, less digestive bloating, better mental focus, more energy, fewer food cravings, or lower blood sugar levels—within a few days of eating totally against the grain. As time goes on, more weight comes off, blood pressure, cholesterol, and triglyceride levels normalize, and other symptoms improve.

If you try the Totally Against-the-Grain Diet for a month and see some improvement in your condition, but the improvement starts to slow after a while, you probably need a little extra help from supplements, such as chromium picolinate, omega-3 fatty acids, zinc, magnesium, alpha-lipoic acid, vitamin E, and vitamin C, which help insulin function more efficiently. (See Chapter 16 for more information on supplements.)

Helpful adjuncts to nutritional treatment include physical activity, stress reduction through various means, and adequate sleep. Physical activity directly improves insulin sensitivity while stress reduction lowers cortisol levels, which in turn should lower insulin levels. People who sleep seven and a half to eight and a half hours a night process carbohydrates more efficiently than those who sleep less. For the best results on the Totally Against-the-Grain Diet, try to address these contributing factors as well.

A Variation for Those Who Don't See Improvement

If you try the Totally Against-the-Grain Diet for two weeks and don't notice any improvement at all in health—or actually gain a few pounds or have symptoms get worse—you may need to restrict both protein and carbohydrates in your diet. In some individuals, protein contributes to elevated insulin levels. Therefore, restricting carbohydrate intake alone isn't enough: protein restriction is also needed. Try cutting the servings of protein in this diet (three to five ounces per meal) in half, and add more omega-3 fish oil supplements and monounsaturated fats, such as olives, olive oil, avocados, macadamia nuts, and almonds, to your diet. Omega-3 and monounsaturated fats do not elevate insulin levels and help to

The Rules for Cheating on This Diet

It's not a good idea to break the rules often on this diet. If you do, you simply won't be able to overcome Syndrome X, Type 2 diabetes, and other insulin-related health problems. For this diet to work, you must be disciplined most of the time.

However, if you do cheat, it's helpful to know the rules of the game. First, keep your carbohydrates very low most of the day by eating just protein and nonstarchy vegetables. When you want to splurge on something, have it after a balanced meat-and-vegetable meal and eat the meal and the food you're splurging on within one hour, no more. It's best not to indulge in grain-based foods, especially wheat-based foods, because they're common triggers for food cravings and overeating.

The following are some of the lowest carbohydrate cheat foods I know of:

Amaretto Protein Bar* or other low-carbohydrate, grain-free protein bars without hydrogenated oil, high-fructose corn syrup, or sugar

Fruit shake with coconut milk, 1 to 2 tablespoons protein powder, a few teaspoons of flaxseed meal, 1 cup or so of frozen berries or chopped pineapple and ice, and a pinch of stevia, stevia with FOS, or SweetBalance

A large bowl of strawberries, raspberries, or sliced peaches with coconut cream or whipped cream sweetened with stevia and vanilla

A large bowl of berries topped with shaved dark chocolate

Brownies made with Fran Gare's Decadent Dessert product (sweetened with xylitol and available through www.frangare.com)

Papadums coated with olive oil and microwaved, served with Guacamole* control the appetite. This variation is often helpful for people with difficult-to-control diabetes.

Moving to a More Moderate Carbohydrate Plan

Continue to follow the Totally Against-the-Grain Diet (or variation) as long as you have overt signs and symptoms of carbohydrate sensitivity. Once your condition dramatically improves, you can make a gradual transition to a more moderate carbohydrate diet, if you desire. The following indicators can tell you if you're ready to do this.

- Your blood pressure, blood cholesterol, and blood triglyceride readings have reached healthy levels and have remained in healthy ranges for a few months.

- You no longer have two or more strong indicators of Syndrome X (overweight, high triglycerides, high cholesterol, and high blood pressure).

- Your blood sugar and blood insulin levels are in healthy ranges, and you have eliminated (with your doctor's permission) any antidiabetic or insulin-sensitizing medicines you may have been taking.

- You have reached, or come within five pounds of, your ideal weight.

Work with your doctor on evaluating these indicators. When they're favorable, start adding more carbohydrates to your diet. First, include an extra serving of nonstarchy vegetables at each meal. If you do okay with that, take the extra serving of nonstarchy vegetables out and replace it with fruit, particularly more berries, plums, peaches, nectarines, apricots, apples, and grapefruit. Next, in place of some of the fruit, try small servings of starchy vegetables, such as sweet potatoes and yams, then legumes and nongluten grains or grain alternatives, such as quinoa or amaranth. The more your insulin sensitivity has improved, the more you can fashion your diet to look like the Gluten-Free Against-the-Grain Diet.

However, if, in the process of adding servings of new foods, you find yourself gaining weight, craving carbohydrates, getting more bloated, or not feeling well in other ways, take those as signs you shouldn't ignore: avoid the foods that are problematic and return to the type and amount of carbohydrates you feel (and look) best eating. Everyone has a different amount of carbohydrates he or she thrives on. It's up to you to determine the level that is best for you.

In the next chapter, you'll learn about the middle-of-the-road diet on the grain spectrum—the Gluten-Free Against-the-Grain diet. It is moderate in carbohydrates and specifically for those with gluten sensitivity.

CHAPTER 13

The Gluten-Free Against-the-Grain Diet and Menu Plan

The Gluten-Free Against-the-Grain Diet avoids all wheat, rye, barley, oats, spelt, kamut, triticale, and additives made from these foods. As in all the against-the-grain diets, it is free of refined sugars and rich in nonstarchy vegetables, protein, and heart-healthy monounsaturated and omega-3 fats. The Gluten-Free Against-the-Grain Diet is right for you if:

- You scored high on the Gluten Sensitivity questionnaire.
- You have celiac disease.
- You have dermatitis herpetiformis (a gluten-dependent, itchy, blistering skin disease).
- You tested positive, through a blood test or stool test, for gluten sensitivity.
- You have any type of unexplained illness that has not been helped through standard means.

The menu I've developed is for most busy North Americans who need to avoid gluten. It includes controlled servings of starchy vegetables and legumes, whole-grain rices, a few other types of unrefined grains, and simple recipes using gluten-free flours.

Characteristics of the
Gluten-Free Against-the-Grain Diet

• Moderate carbohydrate

• Free of gluten grains and refined sugars

• Rich in nonstarchy vegetables

• Rich in protein and monounsaturated and omega-3 fats

The carbohydrates that are emphasized are low-glycemic, nonstarchy vegetables along with small amounts of low-glycemic fruits and nuts. If you're moderately carbohydrate sensitive in addition to being gluten sensitive, it's important to lower the carbohydrate content of this diet by eating nonstarchy vegetables and some fruits and limiting gluten-free grains and other starches. The more carbohydrate sensitive you are, the more your diet should follow the Totally Against-the-Grain Diet guidelines.

Some gluten-sensitive people may do fine with dairy products in their diets. However, sensitivity to cow's milk is quite common among gluten-sensitive people, and it provokes gastrointestinal and other troublesome symptoms. (A strong milk allergy actually can cause damage in the intestinal tract similar to the damage done by gluten in celiac disease.) In addition, gluten-sensitive people with autoimmune disorders, autism, and schizophrenia usually have the best results reversing their conditions by avoiding both dairy products and gluten. For those reasons, the menu plan I've outlined does not contain dairy products (other than as optional ingredients). I suggest you try this diet without dairy for two weeks, and then, if you wish, add some butter and small amounts of cheese and see how you do. If you start to feel bloated or experience gastrointestinal upset or other adverse symptoms, steer clear of dairy foods to promote optimal health.

The menu that follows is one example of how to avoid gluten and load up on vegetables in the diet. It certainly can be modified. As long as you follow the against-the-grain eating guidelines, you can make substitutions whenever necessary, according to your preferences, lifestyle, and sensitivities.

THE GLUTEN-FREE AGAINST-THE-GRAIN DIET PLAN
One-Week Sample Menu

DAY 1

Breakfast	2 poached eggs on ⅔ cup of hash brown potatoes ½ grapefruit
Lunch	Baked sole drizzled with hazelnut oil Roasted Asparagus* Steamed cauliflower
Dinner	Saffron Chicken* ½ cup of brown rice cooked in gluten-free chicken broth Spinach salad with cucumber slices and Fresh Basil Lemon-ette Dressing* or other gluten-free salad dressing
Snack (optional)	Apple slices spread with almond butter

DAY 2

Breakfast	Slice of Nut Protein Bread* *or* a gluten-free flax waffle spread with almond butter and pear slices
Lunch	Small lean broiled steak with grilled onions *or* broiled beef shish kabob with onions and peppers ½ cup of peas Salad of cucumbers, red onions, and tomatoes sprinkled with dill and red wine vinaigrette
Dinner	Baked Mahi-Mahi with Pineapple Salsa* ½ cup forbidden rice or wild rice combination cooked in gluten-free vegetable broth Julienne green beans

Snack (optional)   Leftover Saffron Chicken pieces
                     Cucumber slices

DAY 3

Breakfast   Weekend Ground Turkey Scramble*
                     1 cup homemade fruit salad

Lunch   Tuna tabouli made with chopped parsley, green
                     onion, lemon juice, olive oil, and cooked quinoa
                     in place of couscous

Dinner   Roast turkey breast with sage and natural au jus
                     Baked yam with a dab of nut butter or butter, a
                        few teaspoons of chopped, home-toasted nuts,
                        and a dash of cinnamon
                     Steamed broccoli

Snack (optional)   Handful of home-toasted pecans
                     2 small plums or a nectarine

DAY 4

Breakfast   2 eggs scrambled with spinach and red onions in
                        olive oil, topped with a slice of avocado
                     Sliver of melon or ½ cup of cantaloupe

Lunch   Turkey sandwich with lettuce, red onion slice,
                        avocado slice, and gluten-free condiment of
                        choice on 2 slices of toasted gluten-free bread
                     Carrot and celery sticks

Dinner   Grecian Lamb Balls* with lemon
                     Steamed artichoke with Fresh Basil Lemon-ette
                        Artichoke Dip*
                     Romaine salad with a few pumpkin seeds and
                        Greek olives tossed with Fresh Basil
                        Lemon-ette Dressing*

Snack (optional)   Handful of cashews
Veggie sticks with gluten-free salad dressing or
Fresh Basil Lemon-ette Dressing*

DAY 5

Breakfast   Gluten-free chicken sausage
Baked sweet potato topped with a drizzle of
hazelnut oil or a dab of butter

Lunch   Large spinach salad with a few sliced, reheated
Grecian lamb balls, sliced carrot, and sliced
hearts of palm with hazelnut oil and
balsamic vinegar
Low-sugar, fiber-rich, gluten-free cookie or bread

Dinner   Nut-Coated Pork Chops* with ½ cup
unsweetened applesauce
Baked Onion*
Roasted Asparagus*

Snack (optional)   Handful of macadamia nuts

DAY 6

Breakfast   A few slices leftover meat of any type
Cream of buckwheat cereal or cooked amaranth
with blueberries and a tablespoon of home-
toasted pecans or Hot Quinoa Cereal with
Blueberries and Almond Butter*

Lunch   Large Greek salad with sliced beets, red onion, and
cucumbers, and chicken strips with a dressing
of olive oil, lemon juice, and red wine vinegar
2 microwaved, gluten-free papadums with
hummus

Dinner   Italian shrimp sauté in extra virgin olive oil with
sliced carrot, sliced leeks, sliced hearts of palm,

garlic, spinach, and pine nuts and topped with
chopped fresh basil leaves and fresh lemon
juice and lime juice to taste on ¾ cup baked
spaghetti squash or ½ cup gluten-free brown rice
spaghetti

Snack (optional)   Celery sticks spread with almond butter

DAY 7

Brunch   Caraway Turkey Sausage Patties*
Millet Applesauce Pancakes* *or* Forbidden Rice
    Flour Crepes* *or* Quick Sweet Potato Pancakes*
    topped with sliced nectarine and a dash or two
    of cinnamon

Snack   Bowl of gluten-free chicken vegetable soup
12 grapes or cherries

Dinner   Broiled turkey burger *or* Lime-Marinated
    Turkey Cubes*
Double serving of steamed broccoli, cauliflower,
    and carrots

Snack (optional)   A few olives
Cucumber slices

Sugar-Free Beverage Choices (from best to worst)

Filtered or bottled water, plain or with a lemon or lime wedge

Sparkling mineral water

Unsweetened, gluten-free herbal teas

Plain, unsweetened, unflavored green tea, red bush tea,
    or black tea

Plain coffee without sugar (no more than two cups per day)

Seeing Results

Many gluten-sensitive people start to see some improvements in health—especially signs such as less digestive bloating and upset, less achiness, less depression, and more energy—within a few days to seven days of following this diet. Others, such as those with celiac disease, sometimes require a longer time for the body to heal.

If you have celiac disease without obvious symptoms (in other words, silent celiac disease), it's important to trust the diagnosis you have been given and follow a gluten-free diet for life, even if you don't initially feel a big difference in health. Like all celiacs, you should have periodic blood screenings (and perhaps a biopsy) to confirm that the gluten-free diet is working to heal your gut.

In my opinion, all gluten-sensitive people, not just celiacs, should make the gluten-free diet a diet for life. Not only is this diet the only answer for healing celiac disease, but it also prevents countless gluten-related health complications, such as osteoporosis, small intestine cancer, and autoimmune diseases.

If You See No or Only Partial Improvement

When the gluten-free diet doesn't work, it's usually because people are inadvertently eating gluten without their knowledge, which is sabotaging their recovery. Other reasons for partial or no improvement on a gluten-free diet include other food sensitivities that have not been addressed, nutrient deficiencies, or the need for therapeutic supplements, and unidentified yeast, parasitic, viral, or bacterial infections in the intestinal tract.

If you have celiac disease that isn't healed by a gluten-free diet, it's important to work with your physician to tease out these variables and find the reason for your continuing health problems. Many traditionally trained doctors do not believe in the use of supplements without documented nutrient deficiencies, but I think this is shortsighted: the body uses nutrients to function properly and it can benefit from more nutrients than just those needed to prevent deficiencies (see Chapter 16 for more information on supplements). You might want to talk with your physician about including them in your recovery program, or you might want to see a nutritionist to help you in this area.

If you have mild gluten sensitivity, try the Gluten-Free Against-the-Grain Diet on your own for a month. If you don't notice any improvement in your health, double-check everything you're eating to make sure it's gluten free. If your diet looks clean and you are still having gastrointestinal upset, something other than gluten—for example, dairy foods, yeast, legumes, eggs, gluten-free grains, and food additives—may be causing the trouble. Try a two-week trial eliminating these foods as well as gluten. If you still continue to have serious gastrointestinal symptoms after this experiment, make an appointment with a gastroenterologist or an alternatively minded physician to evaluate the permeability of your gut and the possibility of an underlying infection. The gluten-free diet is very therapeutic, especially when other common allergens are eliminated. If the diet doesn't work for you, it's important to investigate other medical possibilities for your health problems.

A Variation for Those with Serious Autoimmune Disorders

If you have a serious autoimmune disorder (including multiple sclerosis, autoimmune thyroid disease, Type 1 diabetes, rheumatoid arthritis, and Crohn's disease), the gluten-free diet outlined in this chapter may help reduce your symptoms. However, it probably isn't as strong a therapy as you need to give your body the best chance of recovering from your condition.

If you're willing to do whatever it takes to help your body overcome autoimmune ailments, remove not just gluten from your diet, but all grains, legumes (soy, beans, and peas), dairy products, and yeasty foods (bread, cheese, vinegar, mushrooms, and alcohol). When nutritionally treating autoimmune diseases, the goal is to remove all foods that may be triggering your body to attack its own tissues. The relatively new foods in the human diet seem to do that.

Your diet should consist of fish, shellfish, poultry, and meat, lots of nonstarchy vegetables, and small amounts of starchy vegetables (such as sweet potatoes, yams, and winter squash, and perhaps fruits). It's also extremely important for you to greatly increase your intake of anti-inflammatory omega-3 fats by eating more cold-water fish, omega-3-enriched eggs, flaxseeds, and green leafy vegetables and taking omega-3 supplements. Ideally, you should work with a nutritionist who can develop the most therapeutic supplement program for your condition.

It often takes three to six months for this program to begin working. If you feel dramatically better after that time period, you can try reintroducing small amounts of brown rice, wild rice, and other gluten-free grains into your diet. If you seem to tolerate these foods without experiencing a flare-up of symptoms, feel free to add small amounts of these foods to your diet.

In the next chapter, you'll learn about the least strict against-the-grain diet of the three—the Wheat-Free Against-the-Grain Diet. It is designed for people who want to prevent degenerative diseases, people who want to lose weight, and people who are wheat sensitive.

CHAPTER 14

The Wheat-Free Against-the-Grain Diet and Menu Plan

The Wheat-Free Against-the-Grain Diet avoids all wheat, sugar, and refined sweeteners—ingredients that make up a major portion of most North Americans' calorie-dense but nutrient-poor diets. When wheat, sugar, and refined sweeteners are replaced with nonstarchy vegetables, carbohydrates and calories drop to a moderate level. More than half of all Americans are overweight, so this is a good diet for many people to start with, particularly if they don't know where to begin or if they find the other against-the-grain diets overwhelming.

The Wheat-Free Against-the-Grain Diet is right for you if:

- You scored high on the Wheat Sensitivity questionnaire (but didn't score high on the Gluten Sensitivity questionnaire).

- You tested positive, through an IgG antibody blood test, for a food sensitivity to wheat.

- You are overweight and need to lose less than twenty pounds.

- You want to lessen food cravings and get in control of binge-eating.

- You want to prevent heart disease, Type 2 diabetes, and cancer.

Characteristics of the
Wheat-Free Against-the-Grain Diet

- Moderate carbohydrate
- Free of all wheat products and refined sugars
- Rich in nonstarchy vegetables
- Rich in protein and monounsaturated and omega-3 fats

Many people who are sensitive to wheat are sensitive to dairy foods, too, so I designed the menu plan without dairy foods (except as optional additions). You may do fine with dairy products, but I suggest you try this diet as outlined for two weeks. Then try adding a small amount of butter, cheese, or yogurt and evaluate how you feel, not just on the day you try the challenge but for a few days afterward. (Delayed sensitivities can sometimes cause symptoms a few days later.) If you experience digestive bloating or other undesirable symptoms after reintroducing dairy foods, avoid these products to feel your best. If you don't experience unpleasant symptoms, feel free to include them in your diet in moderation.

As with the previous menu plans, this menu is a sample—just one idea of how to put the against-the-grain eating guidelines into practice. Adapt this diet according to your preferences and sensitivities. Just make sure to avoid wheat in all its various forms.

THE WHEAT-FREE AGAINST-THE-GRAIN DIET PLAN
One-Week Sample Menu

DAY 1

Breakfast	1 hard-boiled egg
	½ cup regular cooked oatmeal with ½ apple chopped, a few raisins, 1 to 2 tablespoons chopped pecans, a few teaspoons ground

	flaxmeal and cinnamon *or* Hot Quinoa Cereal with Blueberries and Almond Butter*
Lunch	Beef fajita with no tortilla *or* broiled beef kabob with peppers and onions Large mixed green salad with sliced peppers, radishes, shredded carrot, and sliced black olives with sugar-free red wine vinaigrette
Dinner	Greek Chicken Legs and Thighs* (one leg and one thigh) ⅔ cup brown rice cooked in gluten-free chicken broth Green beans
Snack (optional)	Handful of almonds ⅔ cup fresh or frozen, thawed cherries or grapes

DAY 2

Breakfast	Gluten-free chicken sausage Cream of brown rice or cream of buckwheat hot cereal with slivered almonds, sliced peach, and a dash of cinnamon
Lunch	Broiled turkey burger made with chopped olives and garlic, topped with sautéed red peppers in olive oil Jicama sticks sprinkled with fresh lime juice Large serving Arizona Cole Slaw*
Dinner	Sautéed sole coated in forbidden rice flour or Bhutanese red rice flour Small baked potato *or* ½ cup Greek potato salad, dressed with chopped green onions, chopped fresh parsley, extra virgin olive oil, fresh lemon juice, salt, and pepper

Spinach salad with a few pumpkin seeds, sliced red onion, and gluten-free salad dressing

Snack (optional)   Handful of macadamia nuts

DAY 3

Breakfast   1 or 2 Amaretto Protein Bars* and a bowl of strawberries *or* Breakfast fruit shake with light coconut milk or yogurt, 1 cup frozen strawberries, 1 to 2 tablespoons protein powder of your choice, and a pinch of stevia, stevia with FOS, or SweetBalance

Lunch   Omega Foods salmon burger *or* baked fish of any type with lemon
Double serving steamed broccoli, cauliflower, and carrots

Dinner   Grecian Lamb Balls* *or* broiled lamb chops with herbs
Chopped eggplant, red pepper, shallot, garlic, and pine nuts slowly sautéed in olive oil with a sprinkle of cinnamon
Red leaf lettuce salad with sliced cucumber and sugar-free red wine vinaigrette

Snack (optional)   A few slices leftover meat of any type with mustard or pesto sauce on a rye sourdough cracker

DAY 4

Breakfast   2 poached eggs on 1 slice of toasted 100 percent rye sourdough bread
½ grapefruit

Lunch	Salade nicoise with tuna, hard-boiled egg, cherry tomatoes, sliced olives, slivered, cooked green beans, and a few chopped, cooked potato pieces (optional) on a large bed of salad greens with red wine vinaigrette
Dinner	Lime-Marinated Turkey Cubes* ½ cup brown and wild rice combination *or* quinoa cooked in gluten-free vegetable, chicken, or turkey broth Roasted Asparagus*
Snack (optional)	Celery sticks with cashew butter

DAY 5

Breakfast	Gluten-free flax waffle *or* slice of Nut Protein Bread* spread with almond butter and apple slices
Lunch	Broiled chicken kabob with mushrooms, green peppers, and red onions *or* broiled chicken breast with herbs Large Greek salad with romaine lettuce, sliced beets, cucumber, and red onion, topped with extra virgin olive oil, red wine vinegar, and fresh lemon juice
Dinner	Baked Pork Chops with Caraway Seeds and Cabbage* ⅓ cup unsweetened applesauce Small baked yam or sweet potato with nut butter or butter and cinnamon Steamed broccoli
Snack (optional)	Handful of hazelnuts or pumpkin seeds Plum

DAY 6

Breakfast	Caraway Turkey Sausage Patties*
	Quick Sweet Potato Pancakes* or any
	   low-sugar, wheat-free pancakes topped with
	   1/2 cup unsweetened peach applesauce

Lunch	Salmon with a Hint of Orange and Fennel* *or*
	   broiled salmon with herbs and lemon
	Peas with dill
	Red pepper sticks, celery sticks, and zucchini
	   rounds with hummus

Dinner	Boneless chicken breast pieces in gluten-free,
	   sugar-free pasta sauce on top of Vegetable
	   Spaghetti* or baked spaghetti squash
	Small arugula or red leaf lettuce salad with
	   gluten-free dressing

Snack (optional)	Veggie sticks with hummus

DAY 7

Breakfast	2 eggs scrambled with chopped onions and peppers, topped with a dab of salsa 1 cup of fresh raspberries

Lunch	Leftover chicken in pasta sauce on top of
	   1/2 cup brown rice spaghetti
	Spinach salad with sliced hearts of palm or
	   artichoke hearts, topped with hazelnut oil and
	   balsamic vinegar

Dinner	Shrimp or tofu stir-fry with onions, peppers,
	   Chinese cabbage, shredded carrot, ginger, garlic,
	   sliced water chestnuts, sesame oil, and
	   wheat-free tamari
	1/2 cup brown rice

½ cup cubed fresh pineapple with a tablespoon
of shredded coconut and a dollop of coconut
milk

Snack (optional)   Handful of macadamia nuts

Sugar-Free Beverage Choices (from best to worst)

Filtered or bottled water, plain or with a lemon or lime wedge

Sparkling mineral water

Unsweetened, gluten-free herbal teas

Plain, unsweetened, unflavored green tea, red bush tea,
or black tea

Plain coffee without sugar (no more than two cups per day)

Seeing Results

Most people start to see some improvements in health—say, a loss of a
few pounds or less digestive bloating—within a few days to a week of following the Wheat-Free Against-the-Grain Diet. Glucose tolerance is often
improved quickly, so many people experience better mental focus, stead-
ier moods, and increased energy a few days after beginning the diet.

If you have wheat sensitivity or wheat allergy-addictions, keep in
mind that you may experience adverse symptoms or wheat cravings during the first four or five days on this diet. These withdrawal symptoms
can be uncomfortable, but if you experience them, remind yourself that
they're an encouraging sign (that wheat allergy really is a problem for
you), not a discouraging sign (that the diet doesn't work). Take extra vitamin C with bioflavonoids for a few days to lessen the adverse allergic
symptoms, if you wish; just be sure to keep with the diet for a few more
days. Once wheat gets out of your system, uncomfortable symptoms and
cravings usually dramatically lessen or lift entirely.

As time goes on, the extra nutrient punch of the Wheat-Free Against-
the-Grain Diet builds up nutrient reserves and helps the body function

more efficiently. Minor and major allergic symptoms slough off, and heart-disease and diabetes risk factors—such as extra weight around the middle, elevated blood sugar levels, high blood pressure, high cholesterol, or high blood triglycerides—normalize.

If You See No Improvement or Only Partial Improvement

If you try the Wheat-Free Against-the-Grain Diet for two weeks and notice no or only slight improvement in your health, take a closer look at what you're eating and what symptoms you're experiencing. First, double-check all the foods in your diet to make sure they have no traces of wheat in them. This may seem picky, but if you're wheat sensitive, you might not be able to get rid of your symptoms without removing every trace of wheat in your diet.

If your diet looks completely wheat free, pay attention to the symptoms you're experiencing. If you haven't been able to lose any weight, the diet outlined in this chapter is probably higher in carbohydrates than you need. Cut back your intake of wheat-free grains, starchy vegetables, legumes, and fruits and eat nonstarchy vegetables to your heart's content. Dietary supplements, such as a good multiple vitamin/mineral, extra chromium picolinate, and omega-3 fish oil supplements, can help, too.

If you have digestive upset, the underlying reason for this symptom may be something else you're eating. First, entertain the idea that the culprit may be gluten, not just wheat. Have a gluten sensitivity test performed or try the Gluten-Free Against-the-Grain Diet for a few weeks and see if your digestive symptoms clear up. If this doesn't seem to be the answer, look at other common culprits behind unresolved digestive trouble—for example, hidden yeast overgrowth or sensitivities to milk, soy foods, beans, or corn.

Continuing allergic symptoms, such as asthma, a runny nose, or skin irritations, usually signal that other food sensitivities are involved. The most likely dietary culprits in food sensitivities are foods that you eat repeatedly and foods that are combined with wheat in common American

A Word to Vegetarians

You can adapt the Wheat-Free Against-the-Grain Diet or any of the against-the-grain diets to a vegetarian plan, especially a lacto-ovo-vegetarian plan. To do this, replace the meat, poultry, and fish in the diets with tofu, wheat-free tempeh, eggs (preferably the omega-3-enriched types), dairy products, protein powders, nuts, seeds, nut butters, and perhaps small amounts of beans. Be careful to avoid wheat- and gluten-containing soy-based imitation meats and protein bars and to eat plenty of vegetables. Be aware that some vegetarians can develop sensitivities to protein sources they eat repeatedly, so it's important to vary your diet as much as possible.

If you follow a carefully thought-out vegetarian diet and still experience health problems, it's time to think seriously about modifying your diet. Consider adding small amounts of fish or poultry for the beneficial omega-3 fatty acids and zinc they provide.

foods—such as dairy products, yeast, tomatoes, and corn. Try removing these foods from your diet and see if your symptoms clear up. If you have trouble figuring out which foods are causing problems, invest in an ELISA IgG antibody food-sensitivity blood screen or make an appointment with a nutritionist or nutritionally oriented physician—and try adding supportive supplements to your nutritional program.

Transitioning to a Maintenance Against-the-Grain Diet

If you avoid a problematic food such as wheat for three to six months, you often can add the food back into your diet on an occasional basis without experiencing health problems, according to most allergists. However, wheat contains the highest amount of gluten, and wheat sensitivity can be a precursor to gluten sensitivity. Until more research is done, the jury is still out as to whether reintroducing wheat in the diet might eventually lead to gluten sensitivity and all the health problems that can accompany it.

How much wheat you choose to eat, if any, is, therefore, a matter of personal choice. There isn't a strong nutritional reason to add wheat back into the diet: Refined wheat is a nutrient-poor food, and whole wheat has a lot of antinutrients that can be problematic. The only strong reasons for adding wheat back into the diet are convenience, fitting in with the crowd, and taste. Fortunately, it gets easier and easier to avoid wheat the more you do it, and taste is something that is learned and can change. The more you avoid wheat, the more you will like food without it.

If you try wheat after avoiding it for many months and experience adverse health consequences, you should certainly keep wheat out of your diet. If you don't seem to experience any health problems after reintroducing wheat, resist the urge to eat wheat products frequently and in large amounts—or you will redevelop health problems fast. (I have seen clients over and over again run into this problem. It seems the older people get, and the more health problems they have, the less they can eat wheat without experiencing adverse effects.)

Refined-wheat products act like sugar in the body and should be thought of like dessert—something that should only be indulged in every once in a while. You may be able to get away with eating wheat from time to time, but remember that whole wheat products are poor substitutes for health-promoting vegetables.

If you eat wheat, remind yourself of the information in this book and keep a close eye on your health. If you see subtle signs of wheat sensitivity resurfacing (or other symptoms that could indicate gluten sensitivity or carbohydrate sensitivity), nip the problem in the bud by taking wheat back out of your diet. The nutritional key to staying well for life is to evaluate how far against the grain you need to eat for your best health and to put that information into action.

CHAPTER 15

Recipes

Making up meals that go against the grain may seem daunting at first, but it's really not that difficult, as you'll see in this chapter. With the exception of a few baked goods, the recipes I've compiled here are easy to make and don't involve a lot of fuss.

I tend to be an intuitive cook, adding ingredients to my liking without measuring. Once you start getting the hang of low- to no-grain cooking, I encourage you to do the same. The measurements in these recipes are approximate, and my recipes tend to be fairly forgiving. Feel free to make substitutions or add a little more of one ingredient one day or a little less of it another day. The recipes should still come out fine. They are just good basic recipes or starting points.

The number of people my recipes serve also varies. As a general rule, elderly people tend to eat less, and teenagers and active men tend to eat more. People who are on grain-free, low-carbohydrate diets usually eat bigger portions of meat and vegetables than those who follow moderate-carbohydrate diets that include some grains. I often give a range of servings, such as "serves 2 to 4," to account for different appetites and other variables.

Many of the recipes can be followed by people on any of the against-the-grain diets but some are appropriate for only one or two diets. All the recipes are wheat free. To help you choose which recipes are best for you to use, I've included the following abbreviations next to each recipe: LC = Low Carbohydrate; GrF = Grain Free; GF = Gluten Free.

BREAKFAST FOODS

Hot Quinoa Cereal with Blueberries and Almond Butter (GrF, GF)

1 cup water
$\frac{1}{3}$ cup quinoa flakes
Unrefined sea salt to taste (optional)
$\frac{1}{4}$ cup frozen blueberries
1 tablespoon almond butter or hazelnut butter
$\frac{1}{4}$ teaspoon almond extract (GF, alcohol-free brand, if desired)

Boil the water and add the quinoa flakes and a dash of salt (optional) and cook for 90 seconds, stirring frequently. Remove from the heat and allow it to cool and thicken slightly. Meanwhile, put the blueberries in a small saucepan and heat on low until thawed and warmed. Stir the nut butter into the cooked cereal and mix well until the nut butter is evenly dispersed and no clumps remain. Stir in the almond extract and the thawed blueberries (and resulting blueberry juice). Serves 1.

Joe's Special (scrambled eggs, hamburger, and spinach hash) (LC, GrF, GF)

$\frac{1}{2}$ pound organic lean hamburger
Garlic powder to taste (optional)
4 eggs
2 tablespoons extra-virgin olive oil
2 tablespoons diced shallots or onions
$\frac{1}{2}$ teaspoon basil

½ teaspoon oregano
2 garlic cloves, minced
4 cups fresh baby spinach
   Unrefined sea salt and pepper to taste (optional)

Heat a large nonstick frying pan or wok on medium and crumble the meat into pieces in the pan. Add garlic powder halfway through cooking if desired. While hamburger is cooking, beat the eggs in a small bowl with a fork and set aside. When the meat is browned, take it out of the pan and place on a plate lined with paper towels to soak up excess fat. Drain or wipe away excess fat from pan, then heat olive oil on medium. Add the shallots or onions and herbs and cook for a few minutes, then add the garlic and cook a few minutes more. Add the fresh spinach, toss well to coat, and cook until just wilted. Then add the hamburger and stir everything until well mixed. Pour the eggs over the meat-vegetable mixture and stir gently until cooked to your liking. Taste and adjust seasonings. Serves 2 to 3.

Caraway Turkey Sausage Patties (LC, GrF, GF)

   1 pound organic lean ground turkey
4 to 7 garlic cloves, minced
   1 teaspoon caraway seeds
   1 teaspoon rubbed sage
   1 teaspoon ground fennel
   ½ teaspoon fennel seeds (optional)
   Unrefined sea salt and pepper to taste (optional)

Preheat oven to 350 degrees Fahrenheit. Mix all the ingredients together and shape into 2-inch round sausage patties. Place in shallow baking dish and bake for about 20 minutes. Soak up excess fat with a paper towel, then bake for about 5 more minutes until done. Sprinkle with salt and pepper to taste.

Weekend Ground Turkey Scramble (LC, GrF, GF)

Serve this scramble by itself for a low-carbohydrate breakfast or with melon or a mixed fruit salad for a balanced (and very colorful) way to start your day!

¾ pound organic lean ground turkey
2 tablespoons extra-virgin olive oil
⅔ cup chopped zucchini
⅔ cup chopped red pepper
⅔ cup sliced leeks
4 garlic cloves, minced
¾ teaspoon ground thyme
¼ teaspoon ground sage
   Vegetable, turkey, or chicken broth (optional)
   Unrefined sea salt and pepper to taste
1 tablespoon minced fresh parsley

Crumble ground turkey into a nonstick frying pan and brown until no longer pink in the middle. Transfer ground turkey to a plate lined with paper towels to soak up excess fat. Wipe the frying pan clean, then add olive oil and heat on medium. Add zucchini, red pepper, and leeks. Turn heat to low and slowly sauté the vegetables, stirring often, for about 4 to 5 minutes until done. Add the garlic, and sauté a minute more. Add the ground turkey, thyme, and sage. (If mixture seems too dry, add a tablespoon or two of vegetable, chicken, or turkey broth.) Stir until mixed well and heated through. Add salt and pepper to taste and sprinkle with minced parsley. Serves 2 to 3.

Quick Sweet Potato Pancakes (GF)

These taste more like a bread than pancakes. Save leftovers in the refrigerator: they are good to spread nut butter on.

1 egg (or 1½ teaspoons Ener-G Egg Replacer mixed in
   2 tablespoons water)
1 4-ounce jar organic sweet potato baby food

½ baby food jar of mineral or plain water
1 ½ tablespoons melted and cooled coconut butter or butter
or unrefined hazelnut oil
¾ cup brown rice flour
¼ cup finely chopped pecans
½ teaspoon cinnamon
¼ teaspoon pumpkin pie spice

Preheat a nonstick skillet on medium. Beat the egg with a fork or make the egg replacer, then add the sweet potato baby food. To get all the baby food out of the jar, fill jar half full with water and shake gently with the lid on, then pour contents into the sweet potato and egg mixture. Add melted butter or oil and mix well. Add the brown rice flour, nuts, and spices and mix again. Pour batter into thin, 2-inch pancakes and cook until brown on one side. Reduce heat to medium low, flip the pancakes over, press them down, and cook until done. Serves 2 to 3.

Millet Applesauce Pancakes (GF)

These pancakes are a little sweeter, taste a bit more like traditional pancakes, and should be a hit with the kids.

2 eggs
3 tablespoons melted and cooled coconut butter or
butter or unrefined hazelnut oil
2 cups sugar-free applesauce, peach applesauce, or
other flavor applesauce
1 ½ cups millet flour
½ cup chopped pecans (optional)
Unrefined sea salt to taste (optional)
Cinnamon to taste (optional)

Preheat a nonstick griddle on medium. Mix all the liquid ingredients until well blended. Add to the flour, mix well, then mix in the nuts and cinnamon. Pour batter into thin, 2-inch pancakes and cook on both sides until done. Serves 2 to 3.

LUNCH AND DINNER ENTRÉES

Chicken Legs and Thighs Herbes de Provence (LC, GrF, GF)

3   chicken legs, separated (3 drumsticks and 3 thighs)
1½ teaspoons herbes de Provence
    Water as needed
    Unrefined sea salt and pepper to taste (optional)

Preheat oven to 350 degrees Fahrenheit. Pull back the skin of the chicken pieces and sprinkle crushed herbs over the meat, then pull the skin back to its original position. Place the drumsticks and thighs in a nonmetallic baking pan, add a few tablespoons of water, and sprinkle more herbs over the dish if desired. Bake for 45 to 60 minutes, depending on the size of the pieces. After 20 to 30 minutes, check to make sure there's still water in the bottom of the pan. If it looks too dry, add a few more tablespoons of water. To serve, pull off skin and top with natural au jus. Add salt and pepper to taste. Serves 3 to 4.

Saffron Chicken (LC, GrF, GF)

1½ pounds of boneless chicken breasts
⅓ cup extra-virgin olive oil
6   garlic cloves, finely chopped
¼   teaspoon saffron threads
⅓ cup warm water
    Juice of 2 medium lemons
    Unrefined sea salt to taste (optional)

Cut the chicken breasts into bite-size pieces. Heat the olive oil in a nonstick wok and add the chicken and garlic. Sauté until chicken is done in the middle. Transfer chicken and garlic to a nonmetallic pot. Crush and rub the saffron threads between two of your fingers until they are completely powdered, with no strands remaining. Sprinkle the saffron powder into the warm (but not hot) water and mix until the water turns yellow. Add saffron water into the pot with the chicken and the garlic; add lemon juice and mix. Sprinkle with salt and extra lemon juice at the table if desired. Serves 3 to 5.

Greek Chicken Legs and Thighs (LC, GrF, GF)

3 chicken legs separated (3 drumsticks and 3 thighs)
4 to 6 garlic cloves, finely chopped
½ to 1½ teaspoons oregano
Juice of 1 lemon
1 tablespoon to ¼ cup water
Unrefined sea salt and pepper to taste (optional)

Preheat oven to 350 degrees Fahrenheit. Pull back the skin of the chicken pieces and sprinkle chopped garlic and oregano over the meat, then pull the skin back to its original position. Place in a nonmetallic baking pan. Squeeze lemon juice and sprinkle more oregano over the whole dish, then add water to the pan. (Less water makes a more concentrated sauce; more water makes more sauce, but it isn't quite as flavorful.) Bake for 55 to 70 minutes, depending on the size of the pieces. Halfway through the cooking, check the water level in the pan and add more water if needed. To serve, pull off skin and add extra lemon juice and salt and pepper to taste. Serves 3 to 4.

Lime-Marinated Turkey Cubes (LC, GrF, GF)

I tend to favor simple, tasty meals in which the marinade becomes a sauce for both the entrée and side dishes.

1 pound turkey cutlets
⅓ cup extra-virgin olive oil
Juice of 4 limes
6 small garlic cloves, crushed or minced
1 teaspoon oregano
1 teaspoon basil *or* Spice Hunter Pesto Seasoning
Unrefined sea salt to taste (optional)

Cut turkey cutlets into bite-size cubes and put in a deep, medium-sized, nonmetallic bowl. Preheat oven to 350 degrees Fahrenheit. Add the rest of the ingredients to the bowl, mix well, and let sit for 5 minutes. Pour the turkey and all its marinade into an 8-by-11½-inch nonmetallic baking pan and bake for 25 to 40 minutes. Spoon the cooked marinade over the turkey and serve with vegetables or brown rice. Sprinkle with salt and extra lime juice to taste. Serves 3 to 4.

Filet of Sole Florentine* (LC, GrF, GF)

Here's a light, complete meal in one dish.

4 cups fresh baby spinach leaves
1 tablespoon extra-virgin olive oil
1 cup finely chopped onions
   Grated nutmeg to taste
1 pound sole, flounder, or other mild-tasting fish fillets
   Juice of 1 medium to large lemon
1 teaspoon extra-virgin olive oil
2 tablespoons dill weed or dill-based seasoning (a combination of
   dill weed, onion flakes, lemon peel, and chives)

Wash the spinach well, then steam it for 3 minutes or until wilted. Heat 1 tablespoon olive oil in a nonstick frying pan. Sauté the onions until barely soft, then add the spinach, sprinkle with nutmeg, and stir. Arrange the fish in a single layer over the spinach. Drizzle lightly with lemon juice and 1 teaspoon olive oil, and sprinkle with dill seasoning.

Cover the pan; cook on medium low. Check after 5 to 7 minutes. (Scoop underneath the fish and spinach mixture once to make sure it isn't drying out or burning.) Fish is done when it's milky in color and flakes easily with a fork. Garnish with lemon slices and sprinkle with extra lemon juice if desired. Serves 2 to 4.

*Recipe reprinted, by permission of the publisher, from Jack Challem, Burton Berkson, and Melissa Diane Smith, Syndrome X: The Complete Nutritional Program to Prevent and Reverse Insulin Resistance (New York: John Wiley & Sons, 2000).

Baked Mahi-Mahi with Pineapple Salsa (GrF, GF)

2 mahi-mahi filets
1 tablespoon extra-virgin olive oil
   Ground coriander to taste

SALSA
   1 cup finely chopped fresh pineapple
1 to 2 tablespoons minced green onions or shallots
   3 tablespoons minced fresh cilantro (or more to taste)
1 to 2 tablespoons diced red bell pepper
   Ground coriander to taste
   Cayenne pepper to taste (optional)
   1 teaspoon jalapeño, minced (optional)

Preheat oven to 400 degrees Fahrenheit. Coat mahi-mahi filets and
bottom of baking dish with olive oil and sprinkle ground coriander over
the fish. Cover the dish and bake until done, about 20 to 25 minutes.
While the fish is cooking, mix together the salsa ingredients. When the
fish is done, place it on a serving plate and top with salsa. Serves 2 to 3.

Salmon with a Hint of Orange and Fennel (GrF, GF)

1 pound salmon, filleted into 3 pieces
1 large fennel bulb with leafy top
   Juice of 2 small oranges
2 teaspoons grated orange peel
2 tablespoons extra-virgin olive oil
1 teaspoon unrefined sea salt (optional)
   Chopped fresh fennel leaves, parsley, and chives for garnish
   (optional)

Preheat oven to 400 degrees Fahrenheit and coat a nonmetallic baking pan with olive oil. Mince 2 to 3 tablespoons of the feathery leaves
from the fennel and set aside. Trim off the edges and core of the fennel,

quarter the bulb, cut into thick slices, and put them in the baking pan. Combine the orange juice, orange peel, olive oil, and salt in a small bowl; pour half the juice mixture on the fennel slices. Roast until lightly browned, about 20 minutes, stirring every 5 minutes or so. Take the baking dish out of the oven, push aside the fennel, and place the salmon, skin-side down, in the pan. Brush the salmon with the remaining juice mixture and sprinkle with the minced fennel leaves. Resume roasting until salmon is cooked to taste, about 15 minutes. Serve the salmon with the fennel slices and glaze and sprinkle with parsley and chives if desired. Serves 2 to 4.

Guacamole Shrimp Salad (LC, GrF, GF)

1 cup of frozen salad shrimp
Guacamole (see recipe on page 250)
Lime juice to taste

Put shrimp in a strainer and run water over it to thaw. Mix the thawed shrimp well in the guacamole. Add extra lime juice to taste and serve on baby romaine lettuce leaves. Serves 2.

Grecian Lamb Balls (LC, GrF, GF)

1 pound ground lamb
2 to 5 garlic cloves, finely chopped
2 to 3 tablespoons fresh parsley, finely chopped
2 to 4 teaspoons oregano or mint leaves
2 to 4 teaspoons cinnamon
Unrefined sea salt to taste (optional)
Fresh lemon juice to taste (optional)

Preheat oven to 350 degrees Fahrenheit. In a bowl, knead together the lamb, garlic, parsley, oregano or mint, and cinnamon until they are well mixed. Form into 1-inch meatballs and place in a baking dish. Bake for 20 to 30 minutes until done to your liking. Sprinkle with sea salt and lemon juice before serving. Serves 3 to 4.

Variation

Dill Lamb Balls (LC,GrF, GF)

Substitute 2 teaspoons dried dill for the oregano or mint and omit the cinnamon.

Baked Pork Chops with Caraway Seeds and Cabbage (LC, GrF, GF)

  2 center cut pork chops
  ½ teaspoon extra-virgin olive oil
  4 cups cole slaw cabbage mix from a package or
      finely shredded cabbage
1 to 2 teaspoons caraway seeds
  2 tablespoons or more water
      Unrefined sea salt and pepper to taste (optional)

Preheat oven to 350 degrees Fahrenheit. Heat oil on medium in a nonstick frying pan and quickly brown pork chops on both sides. Put the pork chops in a covered baking dish. Place the shredded cabbage around the pork chops, sprinkle with the caraway seeds, and add 2 tablespoons of water. Bake, covered, for 1 hour. Halfway through, check dish and add more water if needed. When done, sprinkle with salt and pepper to taste before serving. Serves 2.

Nut-Coated Pork Chops (LC, GrF, GF)

  ¼ cup macadamia nuts
  ¼ cup Brazil nuts
  2 center-cut pork chops
  2 tablespoons or more water

Preheat oven to 350 degrees Fahrenheit. Grind nuts in a blender or food processor for 30 seconds until finely ground. Using a spoon, press the nut flour on both sides of the pork chops and place in a covered baking dish. Add a few tablespoons of water to prevent the bottom from burning. Bake, covered, for 1 hour. Serves 2.

LUNCH AND DINNER SIDE DISHES AND OTHER EXTRAS

Roasted Asparagus (LC, GrF, GF)

20 fresh asparagus spears
1 to 2 teaspoons extra-virgin olive oil
    Unrefined sea salt and pepper to taste

Preheat oven to 400 degrees Fahrenheit. Chop the asparagus spears into 3-inch pieces, drizzle olive oil on top, and sprinkle with salt and pepper. Toss to distribute oil well. Roast until tender, about 15 minutes for thin asparagus and 20 minutes for thicker asparagus.

Baked Onion (GrF, GF)

2 medium Spanish onions

Keep skins intact, but brush off any loose dirt. Place in a baking pan and bake at 350 degrees Fahrenheit for 1¼ hours. To serve, remove the outer skins and root ends. Serves 2.

Arizona Cole Slaw (LC, GrF, GF)

3 cups shredded green cabbage
1½ cups shredded red cabbage
½ cup chopped fresh cilantro
2 tablespoons fresh lime juice
¼ cup extra-virgin olive oil
¼ teaspoon ground cumin (optional)
1 to 2 tablespoons chopped avocado, red pepper, or red onion
    (optional)
    Pinch of ground coriander (optional)
    Unrefined sea salt and pepper to taste (optional)

Toss all the ingredients together and season with salt and pepper to taste. Let stand for 15 minutes before serving. Serves 3 to 4.

Vegetable Spaghetti (LC, GrF, GF)

1 carrot
1 medium zucchini or yellow summer squash
1 leek
Small piece of green, red, yellow, or orange bell pepper (optional)
1 to 2 garlic cloves, minced
3 tablespoons extra-virgin olive oil
Unrefined sea salt and pepper to taste (optional)
Shredded fresh basil, chives, or parsley to taste (optional)

Cut the vegetables into very thin, julienne strips about 4 inches long. Heat the oil in a large skillet or wok on medium low. Sauté the carrots for 4 to 5 minutes. Add the remaining vegetables and sauté until they are al dente, about 3 to 5 more minutes. Season with salt and pepper and fresh herbs. Serves 2 to 3.

Fresh Basil Lemon-ette Artichoke Dip and Salad Dressing (LC, GrF, GF)

Here's an all-in-one salad dressing, artichoke dip, or marinade for chicken or turkey breasts.

3 tablespoons extra-virgin olive oil
Juice of ½ small lemon
1 small garlic clove, finely minced
3 tablespoons chopped fresh basil leaves
Unrefined sea salt to taste (optional)
Oregano to taste (optional)

Put all the ingredients in a small covered jar or plastic container and shake well. Adjust the ingredients to taste. (Amount of lemon juice may vary depending on the ripeness of the lemon.) Makes enough for two small artichokes or one medium to large one.

Guacamole (LC, GrF, GF)

This versatile, well-known Mexican dip is good with crudités, papadums, corn tortilla chips, or cooked, chilled shrimp, or as a topping for fish or fajitas.

>   1 large ripe avocado
>   Juice of 1 lime
>   1 to 3 tablespoons finely chopped red pepper
>   1 to 2 tablespoons finely chopped shallot or onion
>   Pinch of ground coriander
>   Chopped fresh cilantro to taste
>   Pinch of cayenne pepper or chili powder, dash of Tabasco
>   sauce, or 1 teaspoon minced jalapeño pepper (optional)

Mash the avocado well with a fork. Mix in the lime juice and the rest of the ingredients. Best if used right after it's made. To store before serving, place plastic wrap directly on the surface and refrigerate to prevent it from discoloring. When used as a dip or topping, serves 2 to 3. Recipe can easily be doubled or tripled.

Nut Protein Bread (GrF, GF)

A protein-rich, grain-free bread that can be eaten as is, used to make sandwiches, or spread with dips, spreads, or nut butters. Can be made plain or with caraway seeds or herbs for more flavor.

>   1 ½ cups raw almonds or hazelnuts or 2 cups raw pecans
>   7 eggs, separated
>   1 teaspoon unrefined sea salt
>   1 teaspoon dried basil leaves, ½ teaspoon each of garlic powder
>   and parsley flakes, or 2 teaspoons caraway seeds (optional)

Preheat oven to 325 degrees Fahrenheit. Lightly grease a jelly roll baking pan. Grind nuts, half a cup at a time, in a food processor. Whip egg whites until stiff. (This works best if done with an electric mixer. If you don't have one, beat vigorously with a whisk or blender; you'll get an acceptable bread but it will be slightly flatter.) In a separate bowl, beat egg yolks, seasonings, and ground nuts together. Beat egg yolk mixture into one-quarter of the whipped egg whites until well blended. Then fold this mixture into the remaining whipped egg whites. Pour into the pan and spread it evenly. Bake 20 minutes or until brown. Allow to cool, then cut into bread-sized slices. Layer slices with parchment paper to prevent the bread from sticking together and store in a covered container. Refrigerate or freeze.

CHEATS AND TREATS

You can enjoy sweet things without the bitter consequences of sugar, wheat, gluten, or grains. All the treats in these recipes are made with nutritious, high-quality ingredients and use sweeteners that are better for you than sugar.

However, no matter how nutritious and free of problematic grains these sweets are, they are still sweets that can contribute to blood sugar problems if overeaten. Therefore, save these recipes for special occasions and, after you indulge in one of these treats, remember to get right back on a low- to moderate-carbohydrate, sugar-free diet.

Amaretto Protein Bars (GrF, GF)

These bars serve nicely as desserts. However, they are packed with protein and good fats, are healthier than commercial protein bars, and can work as quick breakfasts and meals-on-the-go in a pinch. Egg or microprocessed whey protein powder can be substituted for rice protein powder, if tolerated.

2 cups raw almonds (or other nuts)
1 cup rice protein powder or other tolerated protein powder
½ cup flaxseed meal
½ cup sulfite-free macaroon-style coconut or
     ground coconut (optional)
¼ teaspoon Sweet Balance or
     ¼ to ½ teaspoon white stevia powder

$\frac{1}{4}$ teaspoon unrefined sea salt

$\frac{2}{3}$ cup melted and cooled, unrefined coconut butter

$\frac{1}{2}$ cup almond butter (or other nut butter)

1 tablespoon glycerin-based, gluten-free almond extract
   (or other flavoring extracts)

Grind the nuts, half a cup at a time, in a food processor. Melt the co-conut butter in a 350-degree-Fahrenheit oven for a few minutes or over low heat on the stove, then set aside to cool. Mix all the dry ingredients together. Mix the wet ingredients in a separate bowl, then combine with the dry ingredients. Spread a small amount of melted coconut butter over a cookie sheet, cake pan, or 9-by-13-inch pan, then line it with parch-ment paper or wax paper and pat the bar mixture into place. (Note: If you use a cake pan, the bars will be thick and the first one will be harder to get out. If you use a cookie sheet, you can make the bars any thickness you want, but there isn't enough batter to cover the entire cookie sheet; you'll have to create your own edges, which isn't hard to do.) Set overnight in the refrigerator for best results, then score into squares. Can be frozen.

Variations

To this basic recipe, you can experiment with different nuts, nut but-ters, flavorings, and spices according to your taste and what you have on hand.

Apple Cinnamon Almond Protein Bar (GrF, GF)

Add to the basic recipe:

$\frac{1}{4}$ cup unsweetened applesauce

$\frac{1}{4}$ to $\frac{1}{2}$ teaspoon cinnamon

Sweet Potato Almond Protein Bar (GrF, GF)

Add to the basic recipe:

$\frac{1}{4}$ cup sweet potato baby food

$\frac{1}{4}$ to $\frac{1}{2}$ teaspoon pumpkin pie spice

Banana Oatmeal Cookies

Teenagers will love making this easy recipe, which they can share
with their younger siblings.

3 cups old-fashioned rolled oats
1 cup millet flour
1 teaspoon unrefined sea salt
½ teaspoon baking soda
1 teaspoon cinnamon
¼ to ⅓ cup chopped walnuts or other nuts (for better
　　　blood sugar balance) or raisins (for a sweeter taste)
4 medium bananas, mashed
⅔ cup melted butter or coconut butter
　　or ¾ cup unrefined nut oil

Preheat oven to 350 degrees Fahrenheit. Mix dry ingredients in a
bowl. Add remaining ingredients and mix. Drop teaspoonfuls on an oiled
cookie sheet. Bake 15 minutes or until lightly brown on bottom. Makes 3
dozen cookies.

Quinoa-Nut Butter Cookies (GF)

½ cup almond butter, hazelnut butter, or pecan butter
¼ cup unrefined nut oil or coconut butter
　　(liquid at room temperature)
¼ cup honey or maple syrup
1 teaspoon baking soda
1 teaspoon cinnamon
1 cup quinoa flakes
4 teaspoons raisins (optional)

Preheat oven to 350 degrees Fahrenheit. Mix nut butter and wet ingredients together in a bowl. Add baking soda, cinnamon, quinoa flakes,
and raisins and stir well. Drop rounded teaspoonfuls on unoiled cookie
sheet. Check bottoms of soft cookies after 7 minutes. If not brown, cook

for 1 to 3 more minutes. Cool 10 minutes before removing from cookie sheet. Makes 2 dozen cookies.

Peach Clafouti* (GF)

3 tablespoons brown rice flour
1 tablespoon potato starch
½ teaspoon unrefined sea salt
2 large eggs
⅓ cup milk (cow's milk, light coconut milk, nut milk,
     gluten-free rice milk, or soy milk)
2 tablespoons honey, pure maple syrup, or fruit juice concentrate
1 teaspoon vanilla extract (gluten-free, alcohol-free, if desired)
½ teaspoon grated fresh lemon peel
2 tablespoons melted and cooled coconut butter or butter
     A few dashes of cinnamon (optional)
3 cups peaches, cut in 1-inch pieces

Preheat oven to 375 degrees Fahrenheit. Blend all the ingredients except the peaches on high for a minute, or if you don't have a blender, mix well with a wire whisk. The batter will be like a thin pancake batter. Add a dash or two of cinnamon to both the batter and the peaches if desired. Grease two small, ovenproof skillets or pans with coconut butter or oil. Pour and spread a few tablespoons of the batter over the bottom of the pans or skillets and bake in the oven for 5 to 6 minutes. Pull the pans or skillets out of the oven, scoop the fruit on top of the cooked batter, and top with the remaining batter. Bake for 20 to 25 more minutes, or until top is puffy and golden brown. Serve immediately. Serves 4.

*Recipe adapted by permission of the author, from a recipe for Clafouti from Carol Fenster, Special Diet Solutions (Littleton, Colo.: Savory Palate, 1997).

Forbidden Rice Flour Crepes* (GF)

1 cup Lotus Foods forbidden rice flour
1 tablespoon potato starch
¼ teaspoon maple sugar
½ teaspoon unrefined sea salt
½ cup coconut milk
¾ cup water
¼ cup finely chopped pecans (optional)

Mix together all ingredients in a bowl. Preheat a 10-inch nonstick skillet. Pour a scant ¼ cup of the batter onto the skillet and quickly tilt to coat the pan, spreading with a spoon to make a medium-thin pancake. Cook until the edges curl and the underside is golden, about 2 to 3 minutes. Gently turn and cook the underside 2 minutes or until lightly browned. Serve with sliced fresh fruit fillings or toppings and coconut cream or whipped cream sweetened with vanilla and a pinch of stevia, Lo Han fruit concentrate, or honey.

Recipe adapted by permission of Lotus Foods from a recipe for Sizzling Rice Crepes from Lotus Foods.

Variation

You can use the batter to make 2-inch-wide, thin pancakes, which are great with turkey sausage for a festive Sunday or holiday brunch.

Apple Cobbler* (GF)

¾ cup brown rice flour
¼ cup finely ground pecans
¼ to ½ teaspoon unrefined sea salt
¼ teaspoon ground nutmeg
1 teaspoon ground cinnamon
1 teaspoon cream of tartar

¼ cup melted and cooled coconut butter
   or butter or hazelnut oil
½ cup unsweetened applesauce
3 tablespoons pure maple syrup or honey
1 teaspoon baking soda
2 tablespoons boiling water
4 cups baking apples, peeled and thinly sliced
½ cup raisins

Preheat oven to 350 degrees Fahrenheit. Grease a 9- or 10-inch pie pan with oil, coconut butter, or butter. Stir together the first six ingredients in a large bowl. Combine the coconut butter, applesauce, and maple syrup together, then add them to the dry mixture. Add the baking soda to boiling water, stir to dissolve, and add to the batter. Quickly fold in the apples and raisins, then spoon the batter into the pie pan. Bake for 40 to 50 minutes or until pie is brown and apples are tender. Serves 6 to 10 people.

Recipe adapted, by permission of the publisher, from a recipe for Magic Apple Pie from William G. Crook and Marjorie Hurt Jones, The Yeast Connection Cookbook (Jackson, Tenn.: Professional Books, 1989).

Chocolate-Covered Fruit (GrF, GF)

Great for parties or, if you halve the recipe, for intimate anniversary celebrations.

4 ounces unsweetened chocolate squares
1 tablespoon coconut butter or unsalted butter
½ cup unsweetened apple juice concentrate
1 teaspoon vanilla (gluten-free, alcohol-free, if desired)
4 cups fresh fruit (whole strawberries, orange segments,
   or sliced kiwis)

Lightly grease a baking sheet with coconut butter and set aside. With water in the bottom part of a double boiler, turn heat on medium and melt chocolate and coconut butter or butter in the upper part, stirring occasionally. When melted, remove from heat and cool slightly. Mix in juice concentrate a little at a time until chocolate dip is smooth (add a little more than ½ cup if needed for thinner consistency), then add vanilla. Dip and turn ends of fruit into chocolate dip so that the lower half of each piece of fruit is coated, and place on baking sheet. When all the chocolate has been used up, place sheet of fruit in the freezer for 10 minutes to set the chocolate, then move to the refrigerator until ready to serve. Makes 9 servings of 4 pieces each.

Crustless Pumpkin Pie (GrF, GF)

2 teaspoons pumpkin pie spice (or ½ teaspoon each ground ginger, ground nutmeg, ground cloves, and ground cinnamon)
½ teaspoon cinnamon
1½ cups pumpkin puree
3 eggs, beaten
1 cup any type of milk (cow's milk, light coconut milk, nut milk, gluten-free rice milk, or soy milk)
¼ cup honey
2 tablespoons molasses
1 teaspoon vanilla (gluten-free, alcohol-free, if desired)

Preheat oven to 450 degrees Fahrenheit. Add spices to pumpkin puree. In a large bowl, mix together the eggs and milk, then add the pumpkin mixture, sweeteners, and vanilla. Keep stirring until well mixed and smooth. Grease a 10-inch pie pan with coconut butter, butter, or oil and pour in the filling. Bake for 10 minutes, then reduce heat to 350 degrees Fahrenheit and bake about 50 more minutes until done in center. Allow to cool at room temperature, then refrigerate. Best if made the day before eating.

Chocolate Walnut Cake (GrF, GF)

A rich, decadent cake that tastes a lot like brownies when served plain or sprinkled with chopped nuts. For a more festive presentation, top with 100 percent all-fruit raspberry spread and fresh raspberries; whipped cream; or lightly sweetened coconut milk or coconut cream.

2½ cups ground walnuts
½ cup unsweetened cocoa powder
5 large eggs
1 cup maple sugar

Preheat oven to 350 degrees Fahrenheit. Oil an 8-inch nonstick cake pan and line bottom with parchment paper. Mix the ground nuts and cocoa powder with the eggs, one at a time, then slowly add the sugar, making sure everything is mixed well. Spoon the mixture into the cake pan, place on the middle or upper oven rack, and bake for 25 to 35 minutes, until a wooden toothpick inserted into the center comes out clean. Cool for 10 minutes or so, then turn out, remove lining paper, place right side up on a wire rack, and serve. Serves 9.

CHAPTER 16

Supplements to Augment the Against-the-Grain Diets

Y ou get a big nutrient boost when you switch from a typical North American refined-grain diet to any of the three against-the-grain diets. By avoiding grains and emphasizing meats, poultry, fish, vegetables, fruits, nuts, and healthy oils, you get more antioxidants in your diet plus all the B vitamins and lots of minerals in easily absorbable forms (without antinutrients, like those in whole grains). Our nutrient requirements were shaped by a diet rich in animal protein and vegetables, so following an against-the-grain diet will take you very far in giving your body the nutrients it needs for health.

Nevertheless, I recommend the use of nutrient supplements to augment the effects of an against-the-grain diet. Consider that:

- None of us are perfect with our diets every day. One day we may come up short in meeting our zinc needs, another day we might not get enough vitamin B_2. Taking supplements provides extra insurance to meet our daily needs.

- Many of us who have eaten refined grains and refined sweeteners since childhood may have developed subclinical or outright nutrient deficiencies that need to be corrected with supplementation.

- Obtaining adequate nutrients to prevent deficiencies isn't enough to promote optimal health. Taking higher-than-average amounts of nutrients gives the body the building blocks it needs to function more optimally and to overcome our own individual genetic shortcomings.
- Taking digestive aids and nutrient supplements can help correct many types of damage in the body brought about by the use of problematic medicines and a lifetime of unhealthy foods.

Supplements, very simply, work synergistically with the against-the-grain diets to promote better all-around health. Sometimes supplementation can be as simple as taking a once-a-day multiple vitamin/mineral supplement. Other times, supplementation needs to be more extensive, especially when treating serious illnesses. What follows are summaries of the most helpful supplements for protecting and improving health for people with wheat, corn, gluten, or carbohydrate sensitivity.

Basic, Fortifying Nutrients

Fortifying nutrients are the vitamins and minerals that are known to be essential to health. Every nutrient is important, but the following is a quick explanation of the most noteworthy ones for people with grain-related sensitivities.

Antioxidants

The main antioxidants are beta-carotene, vitamin C, and vitamin E: they work synergistically to scavenge hazardous free radicals and reduce damage and aging in the body. People with Syndrome X, Type 2 diabetes, and celiac disease have been found to have excessive levels of free radicals and low levels of protective antioxidants.[1,2] Therefore, people with carbohydrate sensitivity or gluten sensitivity need more antioxidants than people who don't have these conditions.

Carotenoid needs are best met by eating lots of vegetables and fruits. If you want extra insurance, choose a multiple that contains 5,000 to 10,000 IU natural beta-carotene (typically identified as *D. salina* on the label). Natural is also the way to go with vitamin E supplements: look on the label for d-alpha tocopherol or mixed tocopherols with d-alpha tocopherol. A good, heart-protective dose for most people is 400 IU.

To promote well-being and increase resistance to carbohydrate sensitivity and allergies, 500 to 2,000 milligrams (mg) vitamin C daily is recommended. Higher doses (up to 8,000 mg in divided doses throughout the day) are often helpful if you have strong allergy symptoms or if you experience allergic withdrawal symptoms. Keep in mind that most vitamin C is made from corn. If you're extremely sensitive to corn, look for a vitamin C supplement derived from beets or sago palm.

B Vitamins

B vitamins are needed to help your body burn the food you eat efficiently, to make healthy blood, and to support optimal gut, hormonal, immune, and blood vessel function. If you've been eating a high-grain diet, it's likely that you have lower-than-optimal levels of at least one B vitamin. Remember that all grains are devoid of vitamin B_{12}; refined grains are deficient in many B vitamins; and whole grains have antinutrients that interfere with the absorption and metabolism of some B vitamins. To make sure your needs are being met and to help correct nutrient deficiencies from too many grains in the past, try a B-complex vitamin or a multiple that contains 25 to 100 mg of the major B vitamins.

Minerals

A diet high in grains can set people up for deficiencies of zinc, iron, calcium, and possibly magnesium. Zinc and magnesium are critical for supporting optimal insulin function, and zinc helps to heal a leaky gut.[3] Many people, therefore, can benefit from taking a well-rounded multimineral without iron. (Supplemental iron should be avoided unless a deficiency exists because excessive amounts of iron can increase free-radical activity in the body.)

Bone health depends on receiving adequate amounts of not just calcium but also zinc, vitamin C, vitamin D, vitamin B_6, boron, and other trace nutrients. If you have low bone mineral density or osteoporosis, work with a health care professional to fortify bone health from all these nutritional angles.

Chromium

Chromium is the most important mineral supplement to help insulin function more efficiently, yet 90 percent of Americans don't receive adequate amounts in their diets. Therefore, supplementation is a must for just about everyone, especially people who have overindulged in sugar and refined grains or who have carbohydrate sensitivity. Chromium is so effective at reversing insulin resistance that one 1997 study found that 1,000 micrograms (mcg) of chromium picolinate daily completely corrected Type 2 diabetes in patients.[4] Chromium has also been observed to help treat some types of depression and premenstrual syndrome.

For general prevention of carbohydrate sensitivity, 200 mcg of chromium picolinate daily should be sufficient. Higher doses, ranging from 400 to 800 mcg daily, are therapeutic for more severe carbohydrate sensitivity conditions such as Syndrome X and polycystic ovary syndrome. Look for Chromax chromium on labels: it's an indicator of the best absorbed and best utilized form of supplemental chromium.

If you have Type 2 diabetes, start with 200 mcg daily and gradually increase to 1,000 mcg a day. Be careful to monitor your glucose levels closely, though. Chromium works so well at improving insulin function that you will probably need to work with your physician to lower and possibly eliminate any antidiabetic medicines you are taking. Chromium picolinate combined with biotin, listed on labels as Diachrome, is an especially good combination for lowering high blood sugar levels in diabetics.

Healing Supplements

Healing supplements is my umbrella term for: essential nutrients that are not generally found in multiple supplements; vitamin-like, therapeutic substances that are not labeled essential nutrients; and non-nutrient aids that improve digestive function. All these supplements support the body in different ways and help it heal from carbohydrate sensitivity and grain sensitivities.

Essential Fatty Acids

As you learned in Chapter 8, omega-3 essential fatty acids help improve glucose tolerance and reverse insulin resistance. They also lower high blood pressure and high blood triglycerides, protect against heart disease, counter inflammation and autoimmunity (especially in joint diseases, inflammatory bowel disorders, and skin conditions such as psoriasis), and may help to reduce the risk of asthma and allergies. Eating cold-water fish, omega-3-enriched eggs, flaxseeds, and dark green leafy vegetables boosts omega-3 intake adequately for the promotion of good health in many people. If fish doesn't tempt your appetite or if you have any of the above conditions that benefit from higher doses of omega-3 fats, consider taking 1 to 3 grams of EPA- and DHA-rich fish oil supplements daily (or more under the supervision of a health care professional, if you have a serious autoimmune disease).

Gamma-linolenic acid (GLA), found in supplements of borage oil, black currant oil, or evening primrose oil, is another type of fat that can benefit inflammatory conditions such as arthritis and multiple sclerosis. It also can improve high blood cholesterol, diabetic neuropathy (nerve damage), many skin conditions, and premenstrual syndrome. Technically, GLA is a fat the body can make, but the body often doesn't make enough of it because of nutrient deficiencies; excess sugar, alcohol, or trans-fats in the diet; diabetes; hypothyroidism; or viral infections. A good daily therapeutic dose of GLA is 240 to 255 mg daily. As with omega-3 fatty acids, higher doses may be beneficial for the treatment of some autoimmune diseases but should not be taken without supervision.

Alpha-Lipoic Acid and Silymarin (Milk Thistle)

Alpha-lipoic acid, a vitamin-like substance, and silymarin, the active ingredient in the herb milk thistle, are both antioxidants that bolster liver function, lower blood glucose levels, and reverse insulin resistance.[5] One or both of these supplements should be essential components of a supplement plan for correcting carbohydrate sensitivity and are sometimes helpful for people with grain sensitivity. Therapeutic doses range from two to three capsules of standardized milk thistle (such as Nature's Way Thisilyn, which is gluten free) daily and 100 to 600 mg alpha-lipoic acid daily, depending on the severity of the condition. Alpha-lipoic acid combined with GLA is the treatment of choice for diabetic neuropathy.

Glutamine

Glutamine, the most abundant free amino acid in the body, is of utmost importance for maintaining a healthy intestinal lining. Many people can be in short supply because viral infections and major traumas, such as burns, injuries, and surgery, deplete levels of glutamine in the body. Supplemental glutamine is particularly important for people who have inflammatory intestinal disorders, celiac disease, and food allergies. It also helps to curb cravings for alcohol or sugar. Powdered L-glutamine mixed in water is the most affordable way to take the amino acid: therapeutic amounts start at 4 to 5 grams of glutamine powder two to three times a day.

Quercetin

Quercetin, a bioflavonoid found in red and yellow onions, berries, and cherries, is an antihistamine that works with vitamin C to help diminish symptoms of allergies, whether from food, pollen, or other allergens. It's best taken in combination with vitamin C and a high-potency bromelain. A therapeutic dose is 250 mg three to four times daily. This amount can be reduced when allergy symptoms are in control.

MSM

MSM (methylsulfonylmethane), best known for relieving pain in people who have arthritis and other musculoskeletal disorders, is a sulfur-based supplement that also helps relieve allergies in some individuals. The usual dosage for MSM is 1,000 to 5,000 mg in divided doses daily, often in conjunction with vitamin C.

Digestive Aids

Friendly, health-promoting bacteria in the colon, known as probiotics, include lactobacillus acidophilus, bifidobacterium, and bulgaricus. Typically depleted by overuse of antibiotics, friendly bacteria promote good digestion and help stave off and treat diarrhea and other bowel disorders, yeast overgrowth, and food sensitivities. Beneficial bacteria supplements can be found in the refrigerated section of health food stores. Dosages vary from one to twenty billion good bacteria organisms daily, depending on the severity of the condition. A lactobacillus species known as Lactobacillus GG (Culturelle by Vitamin Research Products, 1-800-877-2447) often works well for people who don't respond to supplementation with other beneficial bacteria.

Digestive enzyme supplements, such as hydrochloric acid, pancreatic enzymes, and plant-derived enzymes, come in handy for correcting weak links in digestive function, which, in turn, minimizes food allergies in many people. If you experience gas, bloating, or fullness after meals after you begin eating against the grain, you can try plant-derived enzymes such as fungal enzymes (*Aspergillus oryzae*), papain, or bromelain to see if they help. Betaine-hydrochloride and pancreatic enzymes are valuable for some people, but should only be taken under doctor supervision. Hydrochloric acid in particular should be used cautiously: it can cause ulcers in susceptible people when consumed in excess or not needed. Peptide-splitting enzymes (such as Serenaid by Klaire Laboratories, 1-800-859-8358) may be helpful in minimizing reactions to trace amounts of gluten in some people who have gluten sensitivity or autism.

Developing a Good Supplement Plan

It's best to work with a nutritionist or nutritionally oriented physician to fine-tune a supplement program. If you have celiac disease, for example, you should be routinely tested for deficiencies of nutrients, especially vitamin B_{12}, folic acid, iron, vitamin D, beta-carotene, and zinc, and have your bone mineral density, homocysteine levels, and thyroid function checked.

If you have diabetes or other strong cases of carbohydrate sensitivity, you should have your insulin levels and heart-disease risk factors regularly monitored. By using a doctor to perform tests and get more information on your condition, it's much easier to know which nutrient supplements should be included in your supplement regime for maximum benefit.

A gluten-free multivitamin/multimineral without iron is a general recommendation for most people. (The supplement should be iron free unless you have documented iron deficiency.) Companies such as Carlson and Nature's Life make a number of good gluten-free, hypoallergenic supplements, and Abkit makes AlphaBetic, a gluten-free, once-a-day supplement specifically designed for diabetics. If once-a-day supplements are too low in some nutrients for your needs, try taking a multiple vitamin and a separate multimineral or adding additional single supplements to a gluten-free multiple for more nutritional reinforcement.

If You Have Carbohydrate Sensitivity . . .

The most important supplements for treating carbohydrate sensitivity (some of which can be found in a multiple) are:

Chromium picolinate, 200 to 1,000 mcg daily

Zinc, 15 to 40 mg daily

Magnesium, 400 mg daily

Alpha-lipoic acid, 100 to 600 mg daily, and/or two to three standardized silymarin capsules daily

Antioxidant supplements, especially vitamin C, 500 to 2,000 mg daily, and vitamin E, 400 IU daily

Omega-3 fish oil supplements (with EPA and DHA), 1 to 3 g daily

Taurine, 500 to 2,000 mg daily, and/or biotin, 600 mcg to 4 mg, with chromium picolinate, if blood sugar levels are very high

If You Have Celiac Disease, Gluten Sensitivity, or Other Grain Sensitivities . . .

In addition to a broad-spectrum, gluten-free multiple, the supplements most beneficial for celiac disease, gluten sensitivity, and wheat sensitivity are:

Extra zinc, 25 to 50 mg total per day (or more if under doctor supervision)

Antioxidants, especially vitamin E, 400 IU, and vitamin C, 2,000 mg per day and up, depending on the severity of symptoms, often in conjunction with quercetin and bromelain

Vitamin A (from fish liver oil), an antioxidant that maintains the health of the digestive tract and the immune system, 5,000 to 10,000 IU daily or more if under health care supervision. (Note: if you are pregnant or plan to become pregnant soon, do not take vitamin A, or take no more than 5,000 IU, unless directed by your physician.)

Omega-3 EFA fish oil supplements, 1 to 3 grams daily, and GLA, 240 to 255 mg daily

Glutamine, quercetin, MSM, probiotics, and digestive enzymes as needed

CHAPTER 17

Raising Children
Against the Grain

Eating against the grain on your own can be difficult, but it can be doubly challenging to raise children to eat against the grain. Children, after all, are extremely impressionable and are exposed to peer pressure and advertising pressure galore.

However, parents often go to great lengths to do things for their children that they wouldn't do for themselves. Ask any parents of a child who has celiac disease, and you'll find out that they will move mountains to protect their child from gluten that's hidden in foods. They also will use every trick in the book to teach their child why it's important to identify gluten and steer clear of it so the child can feel his best. I think the same attitude should be adopted by parents of children who have subtle grain sensitivities or parents of children who are carbohydrate sensitive and overweight (which, you'll recall, is an increasingly common problem).

Some people might say it's cruel not to let kids eat the foods they want. I look at it a different way. I think it's cruel (or at least shortsighted) to let kids eat grain-based foods with abandon and be set up for a lifetime of health problems (whether from wheat sensitivity, corn sensitivity, gluten sensitivity, or carbohydrate sensitivity). Don't forget: some children today are developing Type 2 diabetes—a disease of aging—by the time they're ten years old! Diabetes sets the stage for countless complications—

coronary heart disease, stroke, blindness, nerve disorders, kidney disease, cancer, and, in men, impotence. So, letting children eat a lot of junky, grain-based foods "because they're kids" is one of the worst things you can do for your kids' long-term well-being. Health problems from grains start very early in life, so the best thing you can do to establish the foundation for long-term health is to raise children against the grain.

To do that, you need to teach by example, explain the problems with grains simply and clearly to your kids, and be creative about making fun, tasty foods and planning celebratory occasions without problematic grains and excessive sweeteners. This takes patience and perseverance, qualities that all good parents develop to a fine art.

The Serious Nature of
Celiac Disease and Grain Allergy

First things first: Celiac disease or a severe grain allergy are serious conditions that require serious action. If your child has one of these conditions, you probably have already gone through a speeded-up version of what it takes to get your child to eat against the grain. Some examples: Clearing problematic grains out of your house and explaining that certain grains act like sheer poison; continually reminding your child that avoiding these grains will keep him happy and healthy (of course, your child could be a girl, but for the sake of simplicity, masculine pronouns will be used throughout this chapter); and teaching your child to read food labels and to watch out for problematic ingredients and potentially problematic foods at friends' houses and school.

The nature of celiac disease and obvious grain allergies is such that you have to work fast and make the change to an against-the-grain diet quickly to protect your child's health. Children usually are quick to learn to eat against the grain because they don't want to eat food that makes them feel awful.

If you have just recently found out that your child has celiac disease or a strong grain allergy, I suggest contacting a celiac support group, food allergy support group, nutritionist, or counselor to help you deal with the practical and emotional ups and downs of having to change both your lifestyle and your child's so quickly.

The Nature of More Subtle Health Problems

Working with children with carbohydrate sensitivity or subtle grain sensitivity is different. Kids with these conditions have a harder time recognizing that grains are problem foods for them. They don't want to give up these foods. They've grown up with grains and don't want to look weird in the eyes of their friends, who are usually eating high amounts of grains and sugars.

If you're too strict with children's diets too fast—before they can see the benefits of eating fewer grains for themselves—they might rebel. Especially if they're teenagers, they might eat junkier foods than usual when they're away from home, perhaps in spite of your well-meaning actions.

Fortunately, in many cases, you don't have to be quick, dramatic, and radical when changing a child's diet. If your child is slightly overweight or reacts to grains with mild symptoms, the diet-changing process often can be more gradual. This, in turn, will instill good eating habits that will last a lifetime.

Changing Your Child's Eating Habits Gradually

What follows is an action plan for slowly but surely helping your child to modify his eating habits to eat against the grain and enjoy better health. If you are pregnant or have an infant, the best strategies for trying to prevent grain allergy or celiac disease are to breast-feed for the first year of life and to delay the introduction of grains, especially gluten grains, as long as possible in the diet. When you do introduce grains, vary the types you serve, always emphasize vegetables more than grains, and be especially careful to serve wheat infrequently.

Eat Against the Grain as a Family

If both you and your child have been eating a lot of grains for years, it's important to take action against the grain as a family. You really can't expect your child to change his eating habits if you are eating pretzels, pasta, and bread. Children learn from the examples set by parents, so changing long-standing eating habits always works best if it's an all-in-the-family endeavor.

Before you take any action, make a decision how far against the grain you need to go as a family. Begin by evaluating the grain or carbohydrate sensitivity of each family member—use the questionnaires in Chapter 7 (and perhaps the results of medical tests, if needed)—and weigh that information with emotional and social considerations. Then decide how strict or permissive you should be for the overall health and happiness of your child and family.

Every parent will draw the line at different places with a child's diet according to different circumstances. You know your child best, so trust your judgment and start taking action against the grain to the degree that you deem best. Always keep in mind that you can revise your stance on diet later on, if necessary.

General Guidelines for Inside the Home

Begin by getting problematic grains and sweets out of the house and bringing in healthier substitutes and alternatives, such as fresh fruits, vegetables, nuts, seeds, and acceptable cookies or bread. The pace at which you make these changes is a matter of personal choice. Even if you make the changes slowly, you will have a positive impact on your child's eating habits. When you get all or most wheat products out of your house, you know for sure that your child won't be eating these foods at home—and this is a big part of keeping him well.

Soft drinks should not be allowed in the house, and your child should understand why. Instead, have plain sparkling mineral water on hand at home and gradually switch your child over to it. If necessary, introduce sparkling mineral water mixed with fruit juice, then add less and less fruit juice as time goes by. You can also make sugar-free, iced tea or iced herbal tea, and you should always encourage your child to drink a lot of water. Getting kids to switch from soda pop to water and other sugar-free drinks is one of the first dietary changes to address.

Be creative about sneaking healthy foods into your child's diet in kid-friendly forms. For example, chop vegetables very fine and add them into spaghetti sauce or tuna or chicken salad. Make up guacamole (with heart-healthy avocado and veggies) and serve with papadums. (Kids love to watch papadums poof up in the microwave—and adults love them, too!) Have ready-to-eat veggie sticks and serve them with tasty gluten-free dips.

Also, carefully choose your most important battles and stand firm on those issues. For example, if your child is mildly carbohydrate sensitive, tell him he can have mashed potatoes with dinner, *or* corn chips and guacamole, *or* a gluten-free cookie, but only one of these. Then let him choose. By doing this, you accomplish three things. You teach your child, in a very subtle way, that an excessive amount of carbohydrates is not healthy. You set up a situation where you control what he eats, but you also give him some free will. Even if your child isn't initially happy with your either/or policy, that shouldn't matter. A big part of being a parent is doing what's best for your child even if he doesn't always like it.

General Guidelines for Outside the Home

When your child is away from home, it's much more difficult to control what he eats. Some parents—such as parents of a child with celiac disease—do an admirable job of protecting their child by talking with teachers, friends, family, and babysitters and explaining the serious need for their child to avoid problem grains. Parents of children with mild grain-related sensitivities, though, usually don't have to go to such great lengths.

If you do a good job of having your child eat a nutritious, low-grain, low-sugar diet at home, you have laid the groundwork for good health. When you do that, it probably isn't such a bad thing for your child to have a few foods that he doesn't normally eat when he's out with his friends. Socially speaking, it's much easier for him, and if your child is eating well at home, he can likely cheat a bit away from home without adverse repercussions. If you're lucky, your child may begin to prefer the fresher, tastier food you serve at home and may not be as interested in eating a lot of junky food when he's out on his own.

However, if your child goes to camp and gains a lot of weight, or comes back from a long day at school or out with a friend and experiences a dramatic increase in allergy and asthma symptoms, it's time to have a serious talk with him and explain the intimate relationship between the health problems he has and the grains (and perhaps sweets) that he eats. Emphasize the idea that it doesn't matter what everyone else eats—it matters what foods are good or not good for *him*. Be sure to reassure him that if his friends are really friends, they will still like him even if he doesn't always eat what they eat.

It's also important to talk about the easiest ways for your child to eat against the grain when he's out with others. Sometimes saying "no, thanks" is all that is needed when your child's friends offer him something he shouldn't have. If his friends ask him why he isn't eating some cookies, he can handle it a few different ways. He can say, "I don't really care for those" (a white lie), and then get his friends interested in some other activity. He can say, "I prefer these cookies" (yummy, gluten-free cookies that he brings from home and that his friends will become interested in). The better choice, particularly if he is quite sensitive, is for him to say, "I'm allergic to wheat" or "I don't eat wheat because it makes my allergies worse." His friends might initially be surprised by this statement, but then after a short while, they will accept his different eating habits and think nothing of them. To make this process easier on your child, be sure to reinforce his self-esteem often and give him tasty snack foods and occasional sweets to carry around that his friends will like, too.

Parenting teenagers is extra challenging because teenagers have minds of their own and are out to "sow their wild oats." In the rebellious stage they're in (which, by the way, is a natural part of becoming an adult), teenagers sometimes eat wheat-based foods with abandon and drink soft drinks and sometimes alcohol when they're out on their own. You can't control everything they do, but you must make teenage children understand that they are responsible for the health consequences of their actions—whether that means more cavities, more skin breakouts, more weight gain, more allergy symptoms, or other possible repercussions. It's a difficult fact to face as a parent, but it's important to realize that teenagers sometimes need to make mistakes with their diets and in life to learn what's best for them.

General Guidelines for Special Occasions

Special occasions should be just that—special. Whether the occasion is a birthday, holiday, graduation, or any other type of celebration, it's important to think of ways to make the gathering fun and festive without problematic grains. To accomplish this goal, you might let other dietary standards slide just a bit for a day. But, often, you don't have to compromise much. For example, you can make the Chocolate Walnut Cake (see page 258) for a child's birthday party and not tell anyone it's gluten free. Adults or children alike will gobble it up and never know the difference. You might even get comments about how yummy and decadent the cake is.

When coming up with fun ideas for celebrations, think along these lines: Kids tend to like finger food, party food on toothpicks, and food that is fun to make. A real hit at parties is allowing children to choose their own toppings for tacos (this works if your child can tolerate corn). You can also have children select the ingredients they want for kabobs or let them top gluten-free pizza crust with the ingredients of their choice.

For party desserts, a low-sugar choice that kids usually love is berries or other pieces of fruit on toothpicks with some homemade whipped cream to dip their fruit in. Other always-popular choices are cookies: Pamela's wheat-free and gluten-free cookies, found in health food stores across the country, usually go over big. You also might ask your child to choose whatever he wants—his favorite allowable food—for his party.

Do your best to come up with nice, simple food ideas for holidays and parties, but don't go crazy. Keep things in perspective: Food isn't everything. Fun activities and good entertainment are just as important, and caring family and friends are the most important of all. Special occasions are meant for sharing good times and celebrating life, and you should be able to do that, even when you do it against the grain.

Some Final Words

Learning the real scoop on grains is a bit like reading a story in which the character that everyone thinks is a good guy turns out to be a villain that no one suspected. Grains aren't the holier-than-thou health foods people think they are. Our health actually is suffering from eating the types and amounts we eat and we need to cut down our intake—or cut out grains totally—to rebuild our health.

Does it take courage to eat against the grain? Yes. Is it worth it? You bet! Try the two-week challenge and see for yourself. If you're like most people, you will be amazed and elated by how much better you look and feel. Your life will never be the same. Your experience will make you a believer in this off-the-beaten-path way of eating, and you will want to continue to eat against the grain over the long term because you feel so much better.

Why am I so sure? As I've explained many times throughout this book, grains are high in carbohydrates and calories, low in nutrients compared to the calories they provide, and loaded with antinutrients that deter health in countless ways. Vegetables, on the other hand, are low in carbohydrates and calories, rich in nutrients compared to the calories they provide, and well tolerated. It doesn't take a rocket scientist to look at this shocking information and get the picture.

Here's the good news: you now know this information and you can use it to your advantage. You have the power to prevent and reverse countless health problems. Don't think of yourself as a victim because you have grain or carbohydrate sensitivity: think of yourself as a sage who has learned about the harmful effects of grains on health before most of the rest of the world. You have the inside track: the secret to improving and maintaining health is to go against the grain of society and eat against the grain. Now it's time to do just that.

Resources

Web Sites

www.melissadianesmith.com
Information on how to schedule nutrition consultations with me and going-against-the-grain-related information, including how to order books and links to key Web sites.

www.celiaccenter.org
Center for Celiac Research, University of Maryland
Information on research taking place at the center, including the on-going blood screening research program in the United States.

www.celiac.com/safe_forbidden.html
Safe and Forbidden Lists for Gluten-Free Eating
An up-to-date list of foods and additives that are considered safe for celiacs and those that aren't.

www.gluten-free.org
A Gluten-Free Web site Collection
Links to informative articles on gluten-related health problems (including autism, rheumatoid arthritis, multiple sclerosis, irritable bowel syndrome, and candidiasis), gluten-free recipes, and related topics.

www.GFMall.com
Gluten-Free Food Vendor Directory
A thorough list of companies that offer gluten-free (mostly grain- or

bean-based) convenience foods, with links to most of the companies' Web sites.

www.intestinalhealth.org
The Intestinal Health Institute

A nonprofit organization that has a young, enthusiastic, service-oriented staff and is dedicated to improving intestinal and overall health and nutrition through medical research, public service, and education. The institute is a great resource for people with hard-to-treat intestinal disorders.

www.nutritionreporter.com
The Nutrition Reporter Web site

Informative articles on the use of nutrition and dietary supplements.

www.PaleoDiet.com
The Paleolithic Diet Page

Links to articles on the benefits of the Paleolithic Diet, a list of Paleolithic diet–related books, and online support groups.

www.PaleoFood.com
A Web site of recipes based entirely on "PaleoFoods"—meat, fish, fruit, vegetables, nuts, and berries.

www.syndrome-x.com
Information on Syndrome X and the previous book of mine under the same name.

Testing Laboratories

Most testing laboratories prefer to work with physicians. If you can't find a physician to test you for gluten sensitivity, celiac disease, or food allergies, try one of these resources:

Better Health USA
1-800-684-2231
www.betterhealthusa.com

The consumer division of ImmunoLaboratories, Better Health USA offers blood screens for food allergies, gluten sensitivity, celiac disease, and more. The company will send a technician to your home or office to take your blood and have it tested. It sends the results of the test directly to you and offers follow-up support and information.

Dr. Braly's Allergy Relief, the Natural Way
(954) 927-2850
www.drbralyallergyrelief.com

The Web site of allergy specialist James Braly, M.D. Through this site, you can order a laboratory test kit with Dr. Braly's approval for gluten sensitivity and/or celiac disease: it includes preaddressed, prepaid shipping materials and information on where to get blood drawn in your area.

EnteroLab/Finer Health
www.enterolab.com
www.finerhealth.com

Joint Web sites of gluten sensitivity specialist Kenneth Fine, M.D. Through either of these sites, you can order a conduct-at-home stool test for gluten sensitivity, celiac disease, malabsorption, and more. The antigliadin stool test was created by Fine to identify subtle and earlier cases of gluten sensitivity that blood tests tend to miss.

York Nutritional Laboratories
1-888-751-3388
www.yorkallergyusa.com

York Nutritional Laboratories, Inc., is the U.S. division of York Nutritional Laboratories Limited in England, the creators of an innovative, at-home, less expensive IgG ELISA food allergy test. The test, which is endorsed by the British Allergy Foundation, allows consumers to prick a finger for a drop or two of blood, then send it in to be tested for reactions to a wide range of common foods.

Celiac Support Groups

The following celiac support groups in the United States offer eating guidelines, newsletters, periodic local support groups, and national meetings. The Celiac Disease Foundation and the Gluten Intolerance Group recommend the same eating guidelines, which allow for gluten-free grains, such as quinoa, buckwheat, and millet; the Celiac Sprue Association puts greater restrictions on the foods it recommends for celiacs. Call the organizations for information, or check out their Web sites and choose the one that seems best to you.

Celiac Disease Foundation
www.celiac.org
(818) 990-2354

Celiac Sprue Association/USA, Inc.
www.csaceliacs.org
(402) 558-0600

Gluten Intolerance Group of North America
www.gluten.net
(206) 246-6652

Magazines and Newsletters

Sully's Living Without
(847) 835-9760
www.livingwithout.com
A lifestyle guide to support and educate people with food, gluten, and/or chemical sensitivities. This attractive, quarterly magazine has inspirational profiles of people overcoming illness through diet change, food-sensitivity consumer issues, a book review column, information on food-allergy-friendly travel getaways, recipes, and more. The publisher also sells gluten-free dining and shopping cards in three languages.

The Nutrition Reporter

This monthly newsletter summarizes recent research on vitamins, minerals, herbs, and foods. For a sample issue, send a business-size, self-addressed envelope with postage for two ounces, to The Nutrition Reporter, P.O. Box 30246, Tucson, AZ 85751.

Let's Live Magazine

1-800-676-4333

America's oldest, monthly, natural health and preventive medicine magazine. It has solidly researched articles that focus on how diet and supplements help maintain health and reverse disease.

Delicious Living

(303) 998-9390

www.healthwell.com

A complimentary publication distributed by natural food stores. It began as a food magazine for the natural foods industry, but now covers a wide range of natural health topics.

Great Life

1-800-676-4333

Another monthly magazine distributed free of charge in many health food stores. Its articles focus on the use of supplements and diet to promote health.

Natural Health Magazine

1-800-526-8440

Natural Health covers an eclectic range of natural health topics—supplements, herbs, home remedies, diet, food, and lifestyle.

Suggested Health Books

There are many excellent books that provide additional information about the roles of diet, food allergies, celiac disease, carbohydrate sensitivity and supplements in health. Some are described below.

Diabetes: Prevention and Cure by C. Leigh Broadhurst, Ph.D. (New York: Kensington, 1999, $17). An easy-to-read book that offers a wealth of information for those with Type 1 or Type 2 diabetes. It takes a Paleolithic diet and supplement approach to their treatment.

Dr. Braly's Food Allergy and Nutrition Revolution by James Braly, M.D. (New Canaan, Conn.: Keats, 1992, $17.95). A thorough and fascinating guide to food allergies and food addictions.

Food Allergies and Food Intolerance: The Complete Guide to Their Identification and Treatment by Jonathan Brostoff, M.D., and Linda Gamlin (Rochester, Vt.: Healing Arts Press, 2000, $19.95). A comprehensive look at the different ways that certain foods cause problems for some people.

Food Allergy Relief by James Braly, M.D., with Jim Thompson. (Los Angeles: Keats, 2000, $9.95). An easy-to-understand introduction to food allergies, gluten sensitivity, and celiac disease.

Get the Sugar Out by Ann Louise Gittleman, M.S., C.N.S. (New York: Crown Trade Paperbacks, 1996, $11.00). An easy-to-read book that offers 501 consumer-friendly suggestions on how to reduce sugar intake and more than fifty low-sugar, naturally sweetened recipes.

The Protein Power Life Plan by Michael R. Eades, M.D., and Mary Dan Eades, M.D. (New York: Warner Books, 2000, $23.95). A good explanation of how high-carbohydrate diets lead to many degenerative diseases, with an especially informative chapter on the grain connection to autoimmune disorders.

Syndrome X: The Complete Nutritional Program to Prevent and Reverse Insulin Resistance by Jack Challem, Burton Berkson, M.D., Ph.D., and Melissa Diane Smith (New York: John Wiley & Sons, 2000, $24.95; $14.95). The definitive consumer guide to Syndrome X (the combination of insulin resistance with abdominal obesity, high cholesterol, high triglycerides, and high blood pressure), which ages people prematurely and sets the stage for heart disease, Type 2 diabetes, and other degenerative diseases. The book includes therapeutic diets, recipes, and supplement plans for this common condition.

Why Am I Always So Tired? by Ann Louise Gittleman, M.S., C.N.S., with Melissa Diane Smith (San Francisco: Harper San Francisco, 1999, $20; $14). The one and only consumer book on an overlooked health problem in many premenopausal women—copper overload—and the conditions it's associated with, including chronic fatigue, premenstrual syndrome, rollercoaster emotions, panic attacks, and a racing mind.

Why Grassfed Is Best by Jo Robinson (Vashon, Wash.: Vashon Island Press, 2000, $7.50). A short, easy-to-read guide on the surprising nutritional benefits of grass-fed meat, eggs, and dairy products. Also contains a comprehensive list of suppliers of grassfed meat in all fifty states and Canada. Order online at www.eatwild.com.

Companies That Produce and Sell Natural Food Products

The companies and products that follow are by no means a comprehensive list, but they are some of the most helpful that I personally use and recommend to my clients. For more suggestions on healthful convenience products, see the many products mentioned in Chapter 10.

Allergy Resources
(719) 488-3630
1-800-USE-FLAX
A mail-order company that sells a wide selection of natural and allergen-free food and health products, including hard-to-find food items mentioned in this book, such as stevia.

Applegate Farms

(908) 725-5800

www.applegatefarms.com

Manufacturers of high-quality deli meat products that are free of gluten, casein (milk protein), and preservatives. All but a few products are also sugar free.

Casual Gourmet Chicken Burgers and Sausages

(727) 298-8307

www.cgfoods.com

Casual Gourmet makes gluten-free, antibiotic-free frozen chicken burgers and sausages that are a great help for a quick meal when you don't feel like cooking.

Earth Song Whole Foods

(877) 327-8476

www.earthsongwholefoods.com

A small company that makes quality foods based on whole foods, including Grandpa's Secret omega-3-rich, quinoa-based muesli. One version is gluten free, the other is not (it contains oats), and both are enriched with rice protein powder. A great product for use while on the road: just soak the cereal in water, light coconut milk, or any other type of milk.

Lotus Foods

(510) 525-3137

www.lotusfoods.com

www.worldofrice.com

Producers of exotic (gluten-free) rices and rice flour, including forbidden rice, red rice, and kalijira rice. These products make for a nice change from traditional brown rice and can be used to make innovative cuisine.

Mental Processes

1-800-431-4018

www.pumpkorn.com

Mental Processes is the manufacturer of Pumpkorn, a healthy, wheat-free, gluten-free snack food made out of pumpkin seeds.

Northwest Natural

(360) 866-9661

This small but quality-minded company markets gluten-free frozen fish products—salmon burgers, halibut burgers, and tuna with pesto medallions—that are combined with wild rice blends and are suitable only for those without strong carbohydrate sensitivity.

Omega Foods Ltd.

(541) 349-0731

www.omegafoods.net

Makers of low-carbohydrate, gluten-free, dairy-free, frozen salmon burgers and tuna burgers. Convenient to fix, they're suitable for use in any of the against-the-grain diets.

Omega Nutrition

1-800-661-3529

www.omegaflo.com

Omega Nutrition is arguably the producer of the best vegetable oils on the market; the oils are unrefined, organic, and minimally processed. In addition to selling quality oils (which can be shipped directly to your home), the company also is a one-stop shop for other helpful products, such as unrefined coconut butter, stevia, and informative books on stevia, healthy fats, and other nutrition topics of interest.

Pamela's Products

(650) 952-4546

www.pamelasproducts.com

A line of gourmet, wheat-free cookies, all of which are gluten free except the oatmeal cookies. These cookies are so tasty you can feed them to kids and non-gluten-sensitive friends, and they will never know that the cookies don't contain wheat.

Trader Joe's
1-800-746-7857
www.traderjoes.com
A growing chain of specialty retail grocery stores with locations originally along the West and East Coasts of the United States. Trader Joe's buys products directly from suppliers in large volume, so it offers great buys on items such as organic produce, nuts, special canned items, poultry sausages, frozen shrimp, fish, and berries.

Wild Oats
1-800-494-WILD
www.wildoats.com
This nationwide family of natural food stores, including Wild Oats, Alfalfa's, and Nature's Northwest, offers everything supermarkets do, but with an emphasis on organically grown produce, organically produced meat and groceries, and natural foods for special diets.

Whole Foods
www.wholefoods.com
The largest nationwide chain of natural food stores, Whole Foods offers fresh organically produced meats, organic produce, and a wide variety of hypoallergenic food products.

Companies That Sell Vitamins, Minerals, and Herbal Supplements

Supplements from companies that have historically sold their products in health food stores are the best choice because they generally are manufactured without sugar and artificial colorings, and many don't have allergenic ingredients, such as wheat. Always read labels carefully and call the manufacturer when in doubt.

Abkit/NatureWorks

1-800-226-6227

Abkit manufactures and markets Alpha-Betic, a gluten-free, dairy-free, once-daily multivitamin/multimineral supplement designed for diabetics. Unlike nearly all other supplements of this sort, it contains alpha-lipoic acid and chromium. Although the dosages are modest, it is an excellent base supplement for people with insulin resistance, Syndrome X, or diabetes.

J. R. Carlson Laboratories

1-800-323-4141

www.carlsonlabs.com

Carlson Labs is the maker and distributor of a wide range of wheat-free, gluten-free, sugar-free vitamin and mineral supplements, most of which are dairy free, too. The company is especially known for its high-quality, natural vitamin E products, including supplements, creams, ointments, and suppositories.

Nature's Life

(714) 379-6500

www.natlife.com

Makers of high-quality supplements, including many varieties that are free of gluten, dairy, and other common allergens.

L & H Vitamins

1-800-221-1152

This mail order company sells many leading health food brands of supplements at discounted prices.

Nutricology/Allergy Research Group

1-800-545-9960

www.nutricology.com

Nutricology/Allergy Research Group is one of the most original companies in developing useful, hypoallergenic supplements and products such as Herbal Café, a gluten-free coffee substitute.

Nature's Way
(801) 489-1500
www.naturesway.com
Nature's Way has been one of the leading herb supplement companies and makes a particularly fine, gluten-free, milk thistle product by the name of Thisilyn.

Vitamin Shoppe
1-800-223-1216
This mail-order company sells most leading health food brands of supplements discounted by 25 to 30 percent, which can lead to a hefty savings.

Educational Organization

American Academy of Nutrition
1-800-290-4226
www.nutritioneducation.com
Accredited by the Accrediting Commission of the Distance Education and Training Council (DETC), which is recognized as a national accrediting agency by the U.S. Department of Education. The American Academy of Nutrition is a distance-education, nutrition college that offers degree and diploma programs and more than twenty individual college and non-college-level courses on various aspects of nutrition.

Referral Services

Finding a nutritionally oriented health practitioner who is savvy about wheat, gluten, and carbohydrate sensitivity (and food allergies) requires researching your options and asking a lot of questions. The following referral services can help point you in the right direction.

American College for Advancement in Medicine (ACAM)

www.acam.org

Enter your zip code in this Web site to get a referral to a nutritionally oriented doctor in your area.

Find a Nutritionist

www.findaNutritionist.com

Select your state or country on this Web site to find a nutritionally oriented practitioner in your area.

Other Books by Melissa Diane Smith

Syndrome X: The Complete Nutritional Program to Prevent and Reverse Insulin Resistance, Jack Challem, Burton Berkson, M.D., Melissa Diane Smith

User's Guide to Chromium, Melissa Diane Smith

User's Guide to Vitamin E, Jack Challem, Melissa Diane Smith

Why Am I Always So Tired?, Ann Louise Gittleman, M.S., C.N.S., with Melissa Diane Smith

Notes

Chapter 2

1. S. B. Eaton and M. Konner, "Paleolithic nutrition: A consideration of its nature and current implications," *New England Journal of Medicine* 312 (1985): 283–89.
2. L. Cordain et al., "Plant-animal subsistence ratios and macronutrient energy estimations in worldwide hunter-gatherer diets," *American Journal of Clinical Nutrition* 71 (2000): 682–92.
3. Ibid.
4. Personal communication with Loren Cordain, Ph.D., February 24, 2001.
5. L. Cordain, "Cereal grains: Humanity's double-edged sword," *World Review of Nutrition and Dietetics* 84 (1999): 19–73.
6. Personal communication with Laura Johnson-Kelly, M.A., April 4, 2001.
7. L. Cordain, "Cereal grains: Humanity's double-edged sword," presented at the Designs for Health Institute's Advanced Training in Clinical Nutrition, Las Vegas, Nevada, February 24, 2001.
8. Personal interview with Laura Johnson-Kelly, M.A., April 4, 2001.
9. G. Wadley and A. Martin, "The origins of agriculture: A biological perspective and a new hypothesis," *Australian Biologist* 6 (1993): 96–105.
10. L. W. Johnson-Kelly, "Against the grain: Wheat consumption and disease in Neolithic Europe," presented at the American Anthropological Association Annual Meeting in Philadelphia, December 3, 1998.
11. L. W. Johnson-Kelly, "The evolutionary history of celiac disease," presented at the Ninth International Symposium on Celiac Disease, Baltimore, Maryland, August 10–13, 2000.
12. L. Greco, "From the Neolithic revolution to gluten intolerance: Benefits and problems associated with the cultivation of wheat," *Journal of Pediatric Gastroenterology and Nutrition* 24 (1997): S14–S17.
13. Personal interview with Laura Johnson-Kelly, M.A., April 4, 2001.
14. K. J. Carpenter, "The relationship of pellagra to corn and the low availability of niacin in cereals," *Experientia Supplementum* 44 (1983): 197–222.
15. Cordain, "Cereal Grains," 2001.

16. R. J. Williams and D. K. Kalita, eds., *A Physician's Handbook on Orthomolecular Medicine* (New York: Pergamon Press, 1977), 24.
17. R. F. Schmid, *Native Nutrition: Eating According to Ancestral Wisdom* (Rochester, Vt.: Healing Arts Press, 1994).
18. R. J. Williams, *The Wonderful World Within You: Your Inner Internal Environment* (Wichita, Kans.: Bio-Communications Press, 1998), 93.
19. Ibid.
20. E. Schlosser, "Fast-Food Nation, Part One: The True Cost of America's Diet," *Rolling Stone*, September 3, 1998, p. 62.
21. ———, "Meat and Potatoes, Part Two," *Rolling Stone*, November 26, 1998, p. 74.

Chapter 3

1. G. Frost et al., "Insulin sensitivity in women at risk of coronary heart disease and the effect of a low glycemic diet," *Metabolism* 47 (1998): 1245–51.
2. ———, "The effect of low-glycemic carbohydrate on insulin and glucose response in vivo and in vitro in patients with coronary heart disease," *Metabolism* 45 (1996): 669–72.
3. D. J. Jenkins et al., "Low glycemic index foods in the management of hyperlipidemia," *American Journal of Clinical Nutrition* 42 (1985): 604–17.
4. J. Raloff, "The new GI tracts: For preventing heart disease, diets that control insulin are all the buzz," *Science News* 157 (2000): 236–38.
5. S. B. Roberts, "High-glycemic foods, hunger, and obesity: Is there a connection?" *Nutrition Reviews* 58 (2000): 163–69.
6. D. S. Ludwig et al., "High glycemic index foods, overeating, and obesity," *Pediatrics* 103 (1999): E26.
7. T. M. S. Wolever and C. Bolognesi, "Source and amount of carbohydrate affect postprandial glucose and insulin in normal subjects," *Journal of Nutrition* 126 (1996): 2798–806.
8. ———, "Prediction of glucose and insulin responses of normal subjects after consuming mixed meals varying in energy, protein, fat, carbohydrate and glycemic index," *Journal of Nutrition* 126 (1996): 2807–12.
9. S. Fukudome et al., "Effect of gluten exorphin A5 and B5 on the postprandial plasma insulin level in conscious rats," *Life Sciences* 57 (1995): 729–34.
10. R. J. Williams and D. K. Kalita, eds., *A Physician's Handbook on Orthomolecular Medicine* (New York: Pergamon Press, 1977), 27.
11. USDA government report, "U.S. Agriculture—Linking Consumers and Producers: What Do Americans Eat?" at www.usda.govnews/pubs/fbook97/1a.pdf.
12. A. Lev-Ran, "Mitogenic factors accelerate later-age diseases: Insulin as a paradigm," *Mechanisms of Ageing and Development* 102 (1998): 95–113.

13. A. Festa et al., "Chronic subclinical inflammation as part of the insulin re-
    sistance syndrome," *Circulation* 102 (2000): 42–47.
14. L. C. Pickup et al., "NIDDM as a disease of the innate immune system: As-
    sociation of acute-phase reactants and interleukin-6 with metabolic syn-
    drome X," *Diabetologia* 40 (1997): 1286–92.
15. J. S. Yudkin et al., "C-reactive protein in healthy subjects: Associations with
    obesity, insulin resistance, and endothelial dysfunction," *Arteriosclerosis,
    Thrombosis, and Vascular Biology* 19 (1999): 972–78.
16. A. E. Hak et al., "Associations of C-reactive protein with measures of obesity,
    insulin resistance and subclinical atherosclerosis in healthy, middle-aged
    women," *Arteriosclerosis, Thrombosis, and Vascular Biology* 19 (1999):
    1986–91.
17. J. Nestler, "Polycystic ovary syndrome: Sister to Type 2," *Diabetes Forecast*
    (2000): 114, 116.
18. R. P. Stolk et al., "Insulin and cognitive function in an elderly population,"
    Diabetes Care 20 (1997): 792–95.
19. S. Kalmijn et al., "Glucose intolerance, hyperinsulinaemia and cognitive
    function in a general population of elderly men," *Diabetologia* 38 (1995):
    1096–102.
20. J. Kuusisto et al., "Association between features of the insulin resistance syn-
    drome and Alzheimer's disease independently of apolipoprotein E4 pheno-
    type: Cross sectional population based study," *British Medical Journal* 315
    (1997): 1045–49.
21. S. Franceschi et al., "Food groups and the risk of colorectal cancer in Italy,"
    International Journal of Cancer 72 (1997): 56–61.
22. Y. I. Kim, "Diet, lifestyle and colorectal cancer: Is hyperinsulinemia the miss-
    ing link?" *Nutrition Reviews* 56 (1998): 275–79.
23. L. Cordain, "Syndrome X: Just the tip of the hyperinsulinemia iceberg?"
    Medikament 6 (2001): 46–51.
24. A. de Vegt et al., "Relation of impaired fasting and postload glucose with in-
    cident Type 2 diabetes in a Dutch population," *Journal of the American Med-
    ical Association* 285 (2001): 2109–13.
25. A. H. Mokdad et al., "Diabetes trends in the U.S.: 1990–1998," *Diabetes Care*
    23 (2000): 1278–83.
26. R. J. Kuczmarski et al., "Increasing prevalence of overweight among U.S.
    adults: The National Health and Nutrition Examination Surveys, 1960 to
    1991," *Journal of the American Medical Association* 272 (1994): 205-11.

Chapter 4

1. J. Salmeron et al., "Dietary fiber, glycemic load, and the risk of non-
   insulin-dependent diabetes mellitus in women," *Journal of the American Medical Association* 277 (1997): 472–77.

2. D. R. Jacobs, Jr. et al., "Whole-grain intake may reduce the risk of ischemic heart disease death in postmenopausal women: The Iowa Women's Health Study," *American Journal of Clinical Nutrition* 68 (1998): 248–57.
3. R. Crayhon, "The Paleolithic diet and its modern implications: An interview with Loren Cordain, Ph.D.," *Townsend Letter for Doctors & Patients* 184 (1998): 142–47.
4. Cordain,"Cereal grains," 1999.
5. Z. Wolde-Gebriel et al., "Interrelationship between vitamin A, iodine and iron status in schoolchildren in Shoa Region, Central Ethiopa," *British Journal of Nutrition* 70 (1993): 593–607.
6. Cordain, "Cereal Grains," 1999.
7. Ibid.
8. A. Elnour et al., "Endemic goiter with iodine deficiency: A possible role for the consumption of pearl millet in the etiology of endemic goiter," *American Journal of Clinical Nutrition* 71 (2000): 59–66.
9. E. Gaitan et al., "Antithyroid and goitrogenic effects of millet: Role of C-glycosylflavones," *Journal of Clinical Endocrinology & Metabolism* 68 (1989): 707–14.
10. "Millet—A possibly goitrogenic cereal," *Nutrition Reviews* 41 (1983): 113–16.
11. Cordain, "Cereal Grains," 1999.
12. Ibid., 2001.
13. U. S. Barzel, "The skeleton as an ion exchange system: Implications for the role of acid-base imbalance in the genesis of osteoporosis," *Journal of Bone and Mineral Research* 10 (1995): 1431–36.
14. T. Remer and F. Manz, "Potential renal load of foods and its influence on urine pH," *Journal of the American Dietetic Association* 95 (1995): 791–97.
15. T. Zwillich, "Vegetarians told to increase intake of vitamin A," Reuters News Service, January 9, 2001.
16. Cordain, "Cereal Grains," 1999.
17. Ibid.
18. Crayhon, "The Paleolithic diet," 1998.
19. M. Brune, L. Rossander, and L. Hallberg, "Iron absorption: No intestinal adaptation to a high-phytate diet," *American Journal of Clinical Nutrition* 49 (1989): 542–45.
20. A. S. Prasad, "Zinc deficiency in humans: A neglected problem," *Journal of the American College of Nutrition* 17 (1998): 542–43.
21. H. H. Sandstead, "Zinc deficiency: A public health problem?" *American Journal of Diseases of Children* 145 (1991): 853–59.
22. Ibid.
23. Ibid.
24. H. H. Sandstead, "Fiber, phytates, and mineral nutrition," *Nutrition Reviews* 50 (1992): 30–31.

25. Cordain, "Cereal Grains," 1999.
26. Ibid., 2001.
27. A. Pusztai, "Dietary lectins are metabolic signals for the gut and modulate immune and hormone functions," *European Journal of Clinical Nutrition* 47 (1993): 691–99.
28. A. Want et al., "Identification of intact peanut lectin in peripheral venous blood," *Lancet* 352 (1998): 1831–32.
29. L. Cordain et al., "Modulation of immune function by dietary lectins in rheumatoid arthritis," *British Journal of Nutrition* 83 (2000): 207–17.

Chapter 5

1. T. Gerarduzzi et al., "Celiac disease in U.S.A. among risk groups and the general population in U.S.A.," *Journal of Pediatric Gastroenterology and Nutrition* 31 (Suppl) (2000): S29, Abst. #104.
2. G. Meloni et al., "Subclinical coeliac disease in school children from Northern Sardinia," *Lancet* 353 (1999): 37.
3. Gerarduzzi, "Celiac disease in U.S.A," 2000.
4. A. Ventura, G. Magazzu, and L. Greco, "Duration of exposure to gluten and risk for autoimmune disorders in patients with celiac disease," *Gastroenterology* 117 (1999): 297–303.
5. A. Ventura, "Celiac disease and autoimmunity: Who comes first?" presented at the Ninth International Symposium on Celiac Disease, Hunt Valley, Maryland, August 10–13, 2000.
6. C. Sategna-Guidetti et al., "The effects of 1-year gluten withdrawal on bone mass, bone metabolism and nutritional status in newly diagnosed adult coeliac patients," *Alimentary, Pharmacology & Therapeutics* 14 (2000): 35–43.
7. Ibid.
8. S. Mora, G. Weber, and G. Barera, "Effect of gluten-free diet on bone mineral content in growing patients with coeliac disease," *American Journal of Clinical Nutrition* 57 (1993): 224–28.
9. T. Kemppainen et al., "Bone recovery after a gluten-free diet: A 5-year follow-up study," *Bone* 25 (1999): 355–60.
10. G. K. T. Holmes, "Non-malignant complications of coeliac disease," *Acta Paediatrica* 412 (Suppl) (1996): 68–75.
11. K. S. Sher et al., "Infertility, obstetric and gynaecological problems in coeliac sprue," *Digestive Diseases* 12 (1994): 186–90.
12. P. Martinelli et al., "Coeliac disease and unfavorable outcome of pregnancy," *Gut* 46 (2000): 332–35.
13. Ibid.
14. P. Collin et al., "Coeliac disease-associated disorders and survival," *Gut* 35 (1994): 1215–18.

15. A. Ferguson and K. Kingstone, "Coeliac disease and malignancy," *Acta Paediatrica* 412 (Suppl) (1996): 78–81.
16. G. K. T. Holmes et al., "Malignancy in coeliac disease: Effect of a gluten-free diet," *Gut* 30 (1989): 333–38.
17. H. E. Prince, G. L. Norman, and W. L. Binder, "Immunoglobulin A (IgA) deficiency and alternative celiac disease-associated antibodies in sera submitted to a reference laboratory for endomysial IgA testing," *Clinical and Diagnostic Laboratory Immunology* 7 (2000): 192–96.
18. K. Fine et al., "Malabsorption and abnormal small bowel permeability without villous atrophy in adults with serum antigliadin antibody," Intestinal Health Institute, Dallas, Texas.
19. Personal interview with Kenneth Fine, M.D., December 12, 2000.
20. H. Nellen et al., "Treatment of human immunodeficiency virus enteropathy with a gluten-free diet," *Archives of Internal Medicine* 160 (2000): 244.
21. G. Michaelsson et al., "Psoriasis patients with antibodies to gliadin can be improved by a gluten-free diet," *British Journal of Dermatology* 142 (2000): 44–51.
22. M. Hadjivassiliou, A. Gibson, and G. A. B. Davies-Jones, "Does cryptical gluten sensitivity play a part in neurological illness?" *Lancet* 347 (1996): 369–71.
23. P. Collin et al., "Celiac disease, brain atrophy, and dementia," *Neurology* 41 (1991): 372–75.
24. M. Hadjivassiliou et al., "Headaches and CNS white matter abnormalities with gluten sensitivity," *Neurology* 56 (2001): 385–88.
25. G. Gobbi et al., "Coeliac disease, epilepsy, and cerebral calcifications," *Lancet* 340 (1992): 439–43.
26. A. Ventura et al., "Coeliac disease, folic acid deficiency and epilepsy with cerebral calcifications," *Acta Paediatrica Scandinavica* 80 (1991): 559–62.
27. L. Luostarinen, T. Pirttila, and P. Collin, "Coeliac disease presenting with neurological disorders," *European Neurology* 42 (1999): 132–35.
28. K. L. Reichelt and J. Landmark, "Specific antibody increases in schizophrenia," *Biological Psychiatry* 37 (1995): 410–13.
29. R. Cade et al., "Autism and schizophrenia: Intestinal disorders," *Nutritional Neuroscience* 3 (2000): 57–72.
30. A. M. Knivsberg et al., "Autistic syndromes and diet: A follow-up study," *Scandinavian Journal of Educational Research* 39 (1995): 223–26.
31. Cade, "Autism and schizophrenia," 2000.
32. W. H. Reichelt and K. L. Reichelt, "The possible role of peptides from food proteins in diseases of the nervous system," in *Epilepsy and other neurological disorders in coeliac disease*, G. Gobbi et al., eds. (London: John Libbey & Company, 1997), 227–37.
33. F. C. Dohan and J. C. Grasberger, "Relapsed schizophrenics: Earlier dis-

charge from the hospital after cereal-free, milk-free diet," *American Journal of Psychiatry* 130 (1973): 685–88.

34. M. Doherty and R. E. Barry, "Gluten-induced mucosal changes in subjects without overt small-bowel disease," *Lancet* 7 (1981): 517–20.

35. S. Auricchio et al., "Toxicity mechanisms of wheat and other cereals in celiac disease and related enteropathies," *Journal of Pediatric Gastroenterology and Nutrition* 4 (1985): 923–30.

36. Personal communication with Donald D. Kasarda at the U.S. Department of Agriculture Agricultural Research Service, January 16, 2001.

Chapter 6

1. J. Braly, *Dr. Braly's Food Allergy and Nutrition Revolution* (New Canaan, Conn.: Keats Publishing, 1992), 42–43.

2. S. Husby, J. C. Jensenius, and S.-E. Svehag, "Passage of undegraded dietary antigen into the blood of healthy adults," *Scandinavian Journal of Immunology* 22 (1985): 83–92.

3. ———, "Passage of undegraded dietary antigen into the blood of healthy adults: Further characterization of the kinetics of uptake and the size distribution of the antigen," *Scandinavian Journal of Immunology* 24 (1986): 447–55.

4. S. Husby, "Normal immune responses to ingested foods," *Journal of Pediatric Gastroenterology and Nutrition* 30 (Suppl) (2000): S13–S19.

5. G. Fluge and L. Aknes, "Influence of cow's milk proteins and gluten on human duodenal mucosa in organ culture," *Journal of Pediatric Gastroenterology and Nutrition* 11 (1990): 481–88.

6. R. A. Rhodes, H.-H. Tai, and W. Y. Chey, "Impairment of secretin release in celiac sprue," *American Journal of Digestive Diseases* 23 (1978): 833–39.

7. A. Carroccio et al., "Exocrine pancreatic function in children with coeliac disease before and after a gluten free diet," *Gut* 32 (1991): 796–99.

8. Personal interview with James Braly, M.D., December 19, 2000.

9. G. Mamone et al., "Qualitative and quantitative analysis of wheat gluten proteins by liquid chromatography and electrospray and mass spectrometry," *Rapid Communications in Mass Spectrometry* 14 (2000): 897–904.

10. B. B. Buchanan et al., "Thioredoxin-related mitigation of allergic responses to wheat," *Proceedings of the National Academy of Sciences* 94 (1997): 5372–77.

11. C. P. Sandiford et al., "Identification of the major water/salt insoluble wheat proteins involved in cereal hypersensitivity," *Clinical and Experimental Allergy* 10 (1997): 1120–29.

12. R. Sutton et al, "Immunoglobulin E antibodies to ingested cereal flour

components: Studies with sera from subjects with asthma and eczema," *Clinical Allergy* 12 (1982): 63–74.

13. C. Zioudrou, R. A. Streaty, and W. A. Klee, "Opioid peptides derived from food proteins: The exorphins," *Biological Chemistry* 254 (1979): 2446–49.

14. H. Kather and B. Simon, "Opioid peptides and obesity," *Lancet* 2 (1979): 905.

15. G. Wadley and A. Martin, "The origins of agriculture," 1993.

16. C. Hallert, J. Astrom, and G. Sedvall, "Psychic disturbances in adult coeliac disease III: Reduced central monoamine metabolism and signs of depression," *Scandinavian Journal of Gastroenterology* 17 (1982): 25–28.

17. L. G. Darlington, N. W. Ramsey, and J. R. Mansfield, "Placebo-controlled, blind study of dietary manipulation therapy in rheumatoid arthritis," *Lancet* 1 (1986): 236–38.

18. M. Rosenbaum, R. L. Leibel, and J. Hirsch, "Medical progress: Obesity," *The New England Journal of Medicine* 337 (1997): 396–407.

19. J. A. Nordlee et al., "Identification of a Brazil-nut allergen in transgenic soybean," *New England Journal of Medicine* 334 (1996): 688–92.

20. M. Nestle, "Allergies to transgenic foods: Questions of policy," *New England Journal of Medicine* 334 (1996): 726–28.

Chapter 8

1. T. Remer and F. Manz, "Potential renal acid load of foods and its influence on urine pH," *Journal of the American Dietetic Association* 95 (1995): 791–97.

Chapter 16

1. J. Challem, B. Berkson, and M. D. Smith, *Syndrome X: The Complete Nutritional Program to Prevent and Reverse Insulin Resistance* (New York: John Wiley & Sons, 2000).

2. P. Odetti et al., "Oxidative stress in subjects affected by celiac disease," *Free Radical Research* 29 (1998): 17–24.

3. G. C. Sturniolo et al., "Zinc supplementation tightens 'leaky gut' in Crohn's disease," *Inflammatory Bowel Diseases* 7 (2001): 94–98.

4. R. A. Anderson et al., "Elevated intakes of supplemental chromium improve glucose and insulin variables in individuals with Type 2 diabetes," *Diabetes* 46 (1997): 1786–91.

5. Challem, *Syndrome X*, 2000.

Index